Quick
Keto Meals
in 30 Minutes or Less

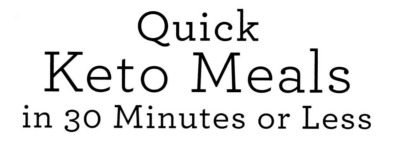

**100 EASY PREP-AND-COOK LOW-CARB RECIPES
FOR MAXIMUM WEIGHT LOSS AND IMPROVED HEALTH**

Martina Slajerova

FAIR WINDS

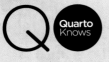

Brimming with creative inspiration, how-to projects, and useful information to enrich your everyday life, Quarto Knows is a favorite destination for those pursuing their interests and passions. Visit our site and dig deeper with our books into your area of interest: Quarto Creates, Quarto Cooks, Quarto Homes, Quarto Lives, Quarto Drives, Quarto Explores, Quarto Gifts, or Quarto Kids.

First published in the United States of America in 2017 by
Fair Winds Press, an imprint of The Quarto Group,
100 Cummings Center, Suite 265-D, Beverly, MA 01915, USA.
T (978) 282-9590 F (978) 283-2742
QuartoKnows.com

Fair Winds Press titles are also available at discount for retail, wholesale, promotional, and bulk purchase. For details, contact the Special Sales Manager by email at specialsales@quarto.com or by mail at The Quarto Group, Attn: Special Sales Manager, 401 Second Avenue North, Suite 310, Minneapolis, MN 55401, USA.

21 20 19 18 17   2 3 4 5 6
ISBN: 978-1-59233-761-3
Digital edition published in 2017

Library of Congress Cataloging-in-Publication Data:
Names: Slajerova, Martina, author.
Title: Keto meals in 30 minutes or less : 100 quick prep-and-cook low-carb
   recipes for maximum weight loss and improved health / Martina Slajerova.
Other titles: Keto meals in thirty minutes or less
Description: Beverly, Massachusetts : Fair Winds Press, [2017]
Identifiers: LCCN 2016049153 | ISBN 9781592337613 (paperback)
Subjects: LCSH: Reducing diets. | Low-carbohydrate diet. | Ketogenic diet. |
   BISAC: COOKING / Health & Healing / Low Carbohydrate. | COOKING / Health &
   Healing / Weight Control. | HEALTH & FITNESS / Weight Loss. | LCGFT: Cookbooks.
Classification: LCC RM222.2 .S5742 2017 | DDC 641.5/6383--dc23
LC record available at https://lccn.loc.gov/2016049153

Design and Page Layout: Amanda Richmond
Photography: Martina Slajerova

Printed in Canada

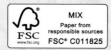

I'D LIKE TO DEDICATE THIS BOOK TO THE AMAZING PEOPLE IN MY LIFE:

To my fiancé, Nikos, who inspires me and makes me laugh every single day. Thanks to you, I was able to pursue the career I've always wanted.

To my family and friends, especially my mom and dad, for their endless love and support. You taught me, challenged me, and always stood by me.

To my grandfather, who will always be the best man in the world. You taught me to be kind and caring and you always believed in me.

Finally, I'd like to dedicate this book to my readers and everyone interested in healthy low-carb eating. I hope my cookbook will help you on your real-food journey!

DISCLAIMER

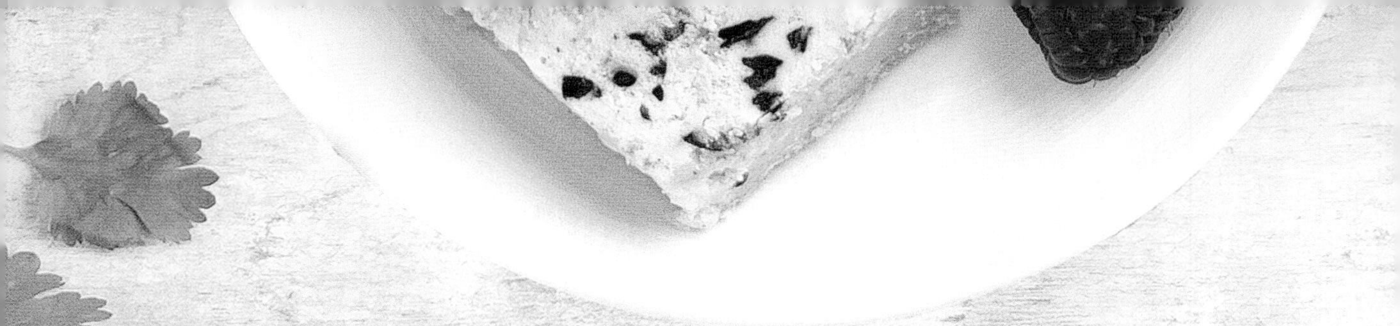

Introduction . . . 7

CHAPTER 1

The KetoQuick Approach . . . 8

Quick Keto Food List . . . 14

An Important Note about Measurements . . . 15

CHAPTER 2

The Basics . . . 18

CHAPTER 3

Breakfast . . . 32

CHAPTER 4

Snacks . . . 56

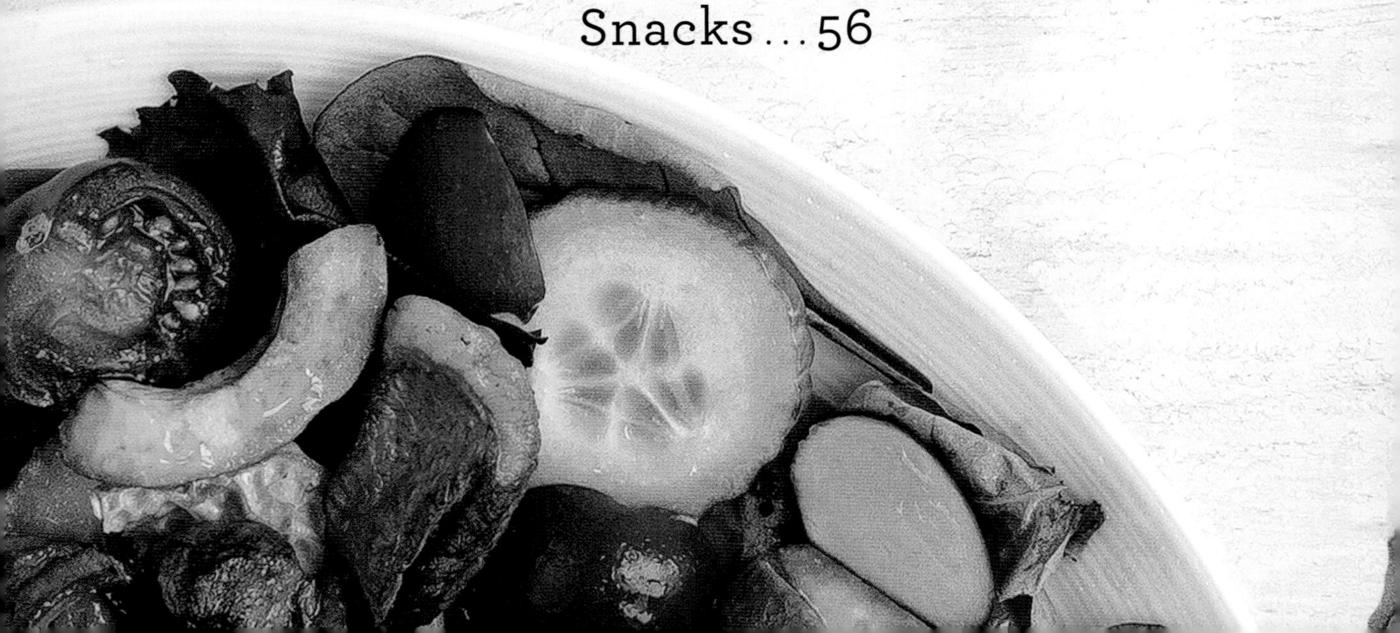

CHAPTER 5

Quick Lunches...66

CHAPTER 6

Soups and Salads...82

CHAPTER 7

Dinner...107

CHAPTER 8

Desserts and Drinks...160

About the Author . . . 186

Acknowledgments . . . 186

Index . . . 187

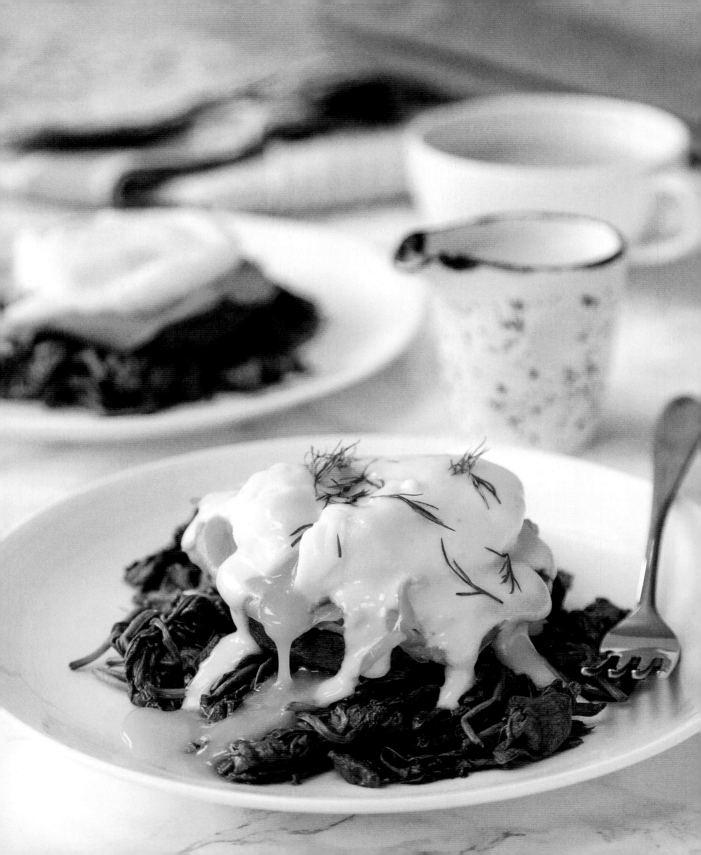

Introduction

As many of you know, I changed the way I ate in 2011 when I was diagnosed with Hashimoto's, an autoimmune disease that affects the thyroid. After my diagnosis, I quit eating grains and sugar, and I started following a primal-friendly ketogenic diet. It wasn't easy at first, but I was tired of following diets that didn't work, and I was determined to regain my health. And it worked! These days, I have more energy to do the things I love, and I enjoy delicious foods that are high in healthy fats. I don't count calories; I exercise less than I used to; and I'm successfully maintaining a healthy weight.

Happily, the days of calorie counting and low-fat diets are over, and it's just a matter of time before the dietary guidelines—which are based on outdated science—change in favor of real, nutritious food.

Not surprisingly, the weight-loss industry has found an opportunity in the obesity epidemic, and has constantly been brainwashing people with advertisements for diet pills, fat-burning shakes, and crash diets that supposedly do the job for us. And, of course, they don't work. I believe that the only effect they have is to contribute to body image issues and eating disorders.

The truth is simple: Healthy eating doesn't have to be complicated, and you don't need to starve to lose weight. When you eat real food that's low in carbs, moderate in protein, and high in fat, you will achieve weight loss by balancing the hormones that control appetite and fat utilization (insulin, ghrelin, and leptin). You simply need to adopt a healthy lifestyle that's also sustainable, so that you'll never feel like "dieting" and depriving yourself of tasty foods. That's what the KetoDiet approach is all about.

Life gets busy, though. If you're like me, you probably don't have hours to spend in the kitchen every day. And that's no problem! This book will show you how to prepare dozens of healthy, delicious, keto-friendly meals—from easy breakfasts to speedy lunches and dinners, plus snacks, beverages, and desserts—all made in thirty minutes or less.

Enjoy!

Martina Slajerova

CHAPTER 1:

The KetoQuick Approach

When I shared my first video recipe on Instagram (@ketodiet_app) in early 2016, I got overwhelmingly positive feedback from people all over the world. I was thrilled! That motivated me to create even more recipes that are quick and easy to prepare—and that's how this cookbook was born.

Eating healthy without spending hours in the kitchen may seem like a challenge at first, but once you learn a few handy tricks and get used to weekly prep routines, you'll realize how much time and money you can save. You'll be able to make tasty, nutritious breakfasts, dinners, and even desserts in just a few minutes. And don't bother looking for a chapter on side dishes in this book, because there isn't one. Thirty minutes or less is all it takes to make a complete meal! Here's how to do it.

1) PREPARE YOUR KETO STAPLES AHEAD.

Cauliflower rice

I like to make cauli-rice in batches. It takes no more than ten minutes, and I don't have to spend time cleaning my food processor when I need it. To make cauli-rice, remove the leaves and the core of the cauliflower. Cut the cauliflower into florets. Wash the florets thoroughly, drain, and pat dry. Once dry, run them through a hand grater or a food processor with a regular blade or a grating blade. (The latter will make the cauliflower look more like rice.) Pulse until the florets resemble grains of rice. Don't overdo it: it takes only a few extra seconds to turn your cauli-rice into cauli purée! Refrigerate in an airtight container for up to 4 days, or freeze for up to 3 months.

Zucchini noodles

Like cauli-rice, zucchini noodles are a great keto-friendly side dish. Wash 2 to 4 zucchini. Use a julienne peeler or a spiralizer to slice them and create thin "noodles." Place in an airtight container and refrigerate uncooked for up to 5 days.

Perfect eggs

Eggs are always on my weekly prep list because they're really convenient when you don't have time to cook. Just throw them into salads or eat with some crispy bacon, smoked salmon, or avocado.

Hard-boiled eggs: Fresh eggs don't peel well. It's better if you use eggs that you bought 7 to 10 days before cooking. Place the eggs in a pot and fill with water, covering them by an inch (2.5 cm). Bring to a boil over high heat. Turn off the heat and cover with a lid. Remove from the burner and keep the eggs covered in the pot (10 to 12 minutes for medium-size eggs; 13 to 14 minutes for large; 15 to 16 minutes for

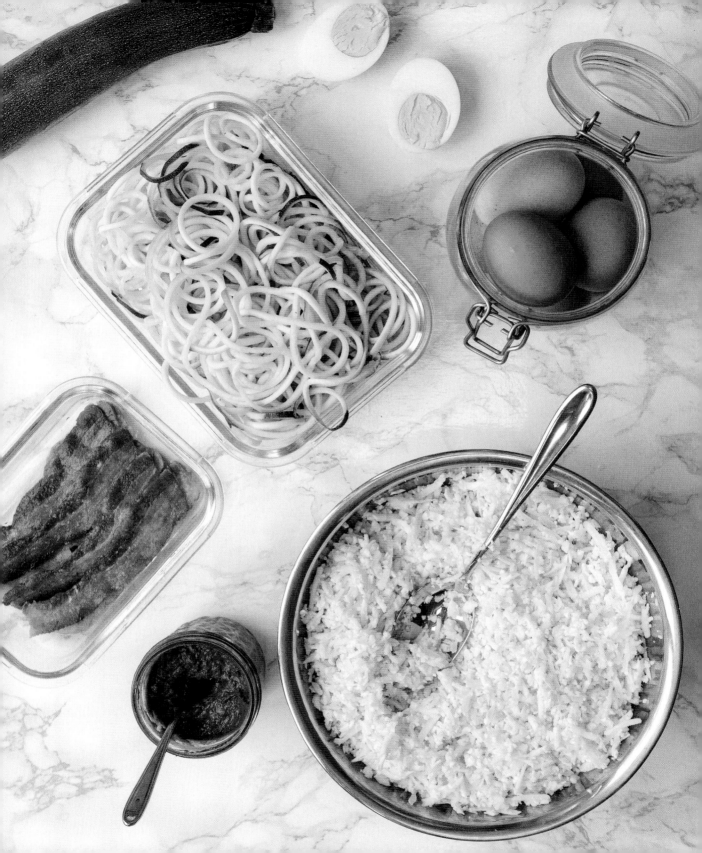

extra-large; 17 to 18 minutes for jumbo and duck eggs). When done, transfer to a bowl filled with ice water and let the eggs sit for 5 minutes. To peel, remove from the ice water and knock each egg several times against the countertop or work surface to crack the shells. Gently peel off the shells. Once cooled, store unpeeled in the fridge for up to a week.

Poached eggs: Fill a medium saucepan with water and a dash of vinegar. Bring to a boil over high heat. Crack each egg individually into a ramekin or a cup. Using a spoon, create a gentle whirlpool in the water; this will help the egg white wrap around the egg yolk. Slowly lower the egg into the water in the center of the whirlpool. Turn off the heat and cook for 3 to 4 minutes. Use a slotted spoon to remove the egg from the water and place it on a plate. Repeat for all remaining eggs. Once cool, place all the eggs in an airtight container filled with cold water and keep refrigerated for up to 5 days. To reheat the eggs, place them in a mug filled with hot tap water for a couple of minutes. This will be enough to warm them up without overcooking.

Fried eggs: Crack the eggs into a large pan greased with some ghee. Cook over medium-high heat until the egg white is opaque and the egg yolk is still runny. As the eggs cook, pour a few tablespoons of the hot fat over the egg whites. Serve immediately. (Fried eggs should not be prepared in advance.)

Crispy bacon
I always keep some crisped-up bacon in the fridge, ready for snacking or for use in a quick salad. (The Ranch Salad in a Jar on page 96 features both hard-boiled eggs and crispy bacon.)

Oven baking: Preheat the oven to 325°F (160°C, or gas mark 3). Line a baking tray with parchment paper. Lay the bacon strips out flat in a single layer, or lay on a wire rack set on top of the parchment. Place the tray in the oven and cook for about 25 to 30 minutes. Remove the tray from the oven and let cool for 5 minutes. Strain the bacon grease into a small jar. Let the bacon slices cool completely and store them in an airtight container in the fridge. Use within 1 week or freeze for up to 3 months.

Pan-roasting: Place the bacon strips in a large pan and add ½ cup (120 ml) water. Cook over medium-high heat until the water starts to boil. Reduce the heat to medium and cook until the water evaporates and the bacon fat is rendered. Reduce the heat to low and cook until the bacon is lightly browned and crispy. Let it cool slightly and cut it into pieces.

Activated nuts and seeds
I buy nuts and seeds in bulk, and I always soak and dehydrate them. Activated nuts and seeds are more easily digested, and their nutrients are better absorbed. Plus, activating makes them deliciously crunchy. To do this, place the nuts or seeds in a bowl filled with water or salted water. Leave at room temperature overnight. Drain and spread on a parchment-lined baking sheet. Place in the oven and dry at a low temperature, or use a dehydrator and dry nuts for 12 to 24 hours, turning occasionally, until completely dry. Store activated nuts and seeds in an airtight container.

Creamed coconut milk
You can either buy ready-made coconut cream or make your own using canned coconut milk. Creamed coconut milk (coconut cream) is the fatty part of coconut milk that has been

separated. If a recipe calls for creamed coconut milk, make it a day ahead. To cream coconut milk, simply place the can in the fridge overnight. Open it the next day; do not shake before opening the can. Spoon out the solidified coconut milk and discard the liquids. One 13.5-ounce (400 ml) can will yield about 7 ounces (200 g) of coconut cream.

2) CHOP AND REFRIGERATE VEGETABLES.

If you don't have time to cook every day, chop your vegetables in advance and keep them in resealable plastic bags or airtight containers in the fridge for 3 to 5 days. That way, they're ready to be used in salads, stir-fries, and other recipes. I pre-cut peppers, onion, cucumber, and zucchini. I prefer to chop soft vegetables (like tomatoes) and any vegetables and fruits that can get discolored (such as eggplant and avocado) just before serving.

3) PARBOIL AND FREEZE VEGETABLES.

Parboiled vegetables take very little time to cook and they stay fresh for longer. To parboil, you'll first buy fresh, in-season vegetables, and then blanch them until half-done but still crispy. To do that, fill a saucepan with water and bring to a boil. Add the vegetables and cook briefly. Exact cooking time depends on the vegetables: less than 1 minute for spinach and chard; 1 minute for asparagus and kale; 2 to 3 minutes for firm vegetables such as broccoli, cauliflower, and green beans.

Rinse the vegetables in ice water and drain thoroughly before placing them in the freezer. I use zip-top bags and divide the vegetables into manageable portions. When you're ready to use the vegetables, defrost them and finish cooking them. Again, the exact cooking time depends on the type of vegetable.

SOAKING TIMES FOR YOUR FAVORITE NUTS AND SEEDS

ALMONDS: Soak for 8 to 12 hours. Dehydrate at 120 to 150°F (50 to 65°C).

HAZELNUTS: Soak for 8 to 12 hours. Dehydrate at 120 to 150°F (50 to 65°C).

PINE NUTS: Soak for 4 to 8 hours. Dehydrate at 120 to 150°F (50 to 65°C).

WALNUTS: Soak for 4 to 8 hours. Dehydrate at 120 to 150°F (50 to 65°C).

PECANS: Soak for 4 to 8 hours. Dehydrate at 120 to 150°F (50 to 65°C).

BRAZIL NUTS: Soak for 4 to 8 hours. Dehydrate at 120 to 150°F (50 to 65°C).

MACADAMIAS: Soak for 4 to 8 hours. Dehydrate at 120 to 150°F (50 to 65°C).

CASHEWS: Soak for 2 to 3 hours. Dehydrate at 200 to 250°F (90 to 120°C).

PISTACHIOS: Soak for 2 to 3 hours. Dehydrate at 200 to 250°F (90 to 120°C).

PUMPKIN SEEDS (hulled): Soak for 4 to 8 hours. Dehydrate at 120 to 150°F (50 to 65°C).

SUNFLOWER SEEDS (hulled): Soak for 4 to 8 hours. Dehydrate at 120 to 150°F (50 to 65°C).

SESAME SEEDS (hulled): Soak for 4 to 8 hours. Dehydrate at 120 to 150°F (50 to 65°C).

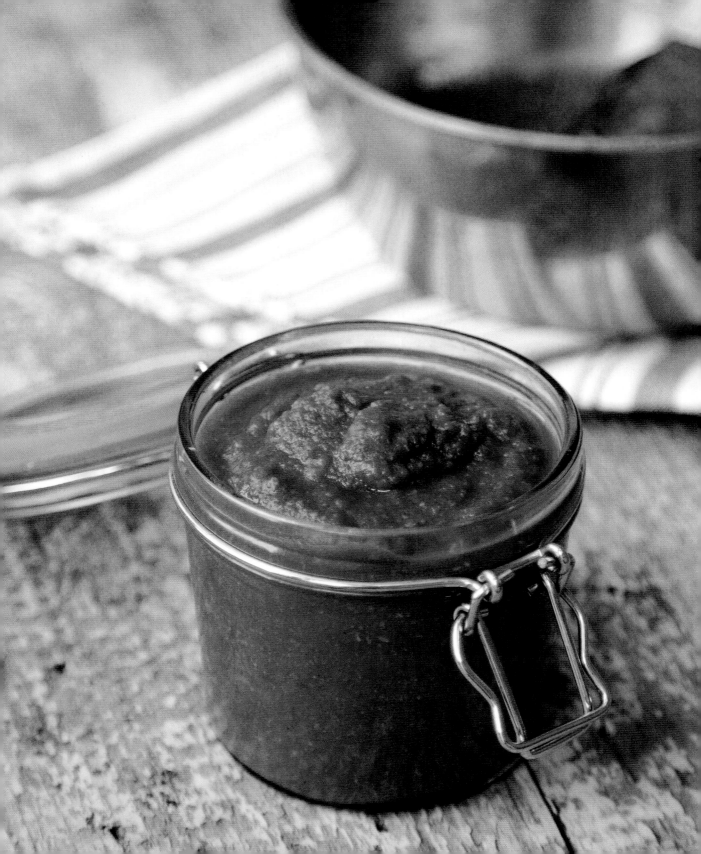

4) FREEZE BERRIES AND HERBS.

Fresh berries last for only a few days, so place them in resealable plastic bags and freeze for up to 3 months. Apart from freezing berries, you can preserve them by making chia jams like Raspberry Chia Jam (page 29).

If you don't have space to keep pots of herbs, you can store cut herbs in several ways: frozen into ice cubes; chopped and frozen in resealable freezer bags; or with healthy fats—as pesto, for instance.

5) MEASURE DRY INGREDIENTS AHEAD OF TIME.

Mix up frequently used dry ingredients, such as baking mixes or spices, in advance. Place them in resealable plastic bags or containers, and use as needed. (Don't forget to label the container.)

6) MARINATE FISH AND MEAT OVERNIGHT.

Marinating is a great way to prepare meat and fish. It adds flavor and reduces cooking time by up to a third. Marinate fish for 2 to 6 hours, and meat for up to 24 hours. Simply place in a resealable plastic bag or container with a marinade made from extra-virgin olive oil, herbs, spices, and lemon juice or vinegar. (The acidic ingredient reduces the cooking time.)

7) MAKE YOUR OWN CONDIMENTS.

I make my own mustard, ketchup, bone broth, pesto, ghee, mayo, pumpkin purée, harissa paste, Sriracha, and more. Why? Making condiments is less expensive and gives you complete control over the ingredients. And the results are so much tastier than store-bought. Learn how to make most keto cooking staples at www.ketodietapp.com/blog.

8) SLOW DOWN.

Getting a slow cooker or a pressure cooker will save you time and money because it'll let you cook meat and vegetables for the whole week with minimum hands-on time. Another advantage is that you can use cheaper, nutritious meat cuts, such as beef brisket or pork shoulder, which are perfect for slow cooking. You can use slow-cooked meat in salads, in wraps, or on top of omelets, or simply eat it with a side of cooked vegetables.

9) MAKE BONE BROTH, CHICKEN STOCK, OR VEGETABLE STOCK.

I use bone broth or chicken stock almost daily, so I make a batch every week. Making broth is easy: Keep leftover bones in a freezer bag until you have enough to fill about two-thirds of your slow cooker. Then, simply throw them into the slow cooker, add your choice of spices, fresh or dried herbs, vegetables, and enough water to cover everything. Cook for 12 to 24 hours. (If you use a pressure cooker, you can make broth or stock in less than an hour.) For vegetable stock, use leftover vegetables such as celery, carrots, onion, garlic, and herbs.

My favorite version of bone broth is a meaty one. To make it, place a whole chicken or oxtails in a slow cooker, add enough water to cover, and cook until the meat is tender and falls off the bones. Remove the chicken or oxtails from the stock. When cool enough to handle, remove the meat from the bones and reserve for use in quick salads or wraps. Return the bones to the stock. Add more bones if you have any in the freezer, plus vegetables and dried herbs of your choice, salt, and a splash of lemon juice. Continue to cook for 12 to 24 hours, strain, discard the solids, and cool. Refrigerate, or freeze the broth in small containers or ice cube trays.

10) USE LEFTOVERS.

Food waste doesn't just affect your wallet; it's a global issue because it contributes to environmental damage and increased carbon emissions. Surprisingly, it's not the supermarkets or farmers who are wasting the most food. It's us, the consumers! So, minimize food waste by always using leftovers.

- When you slow cook meat, use the leftover gravy to sauté your vegetables. It adds flavor, and nothing goes to waste.

- How about the meat from last night's dinner? Turn it into tomorrow's lunch. Add it to your lunch box with vegetables, or wrap in some chard leaves for a low-carb "sandwich."

- Use vegetable scraps such as celery ends, kale stems, and herb stems for making bone broth or vegetable stock. Keep them in a freezer bag until you have enough to make a batch.

- Did you know that peeled broccoli or cauliflower stems are deliciously crispy and perfect for dipping—just like carrot sticks? Try them with Easy Chicken Liver Pâté (page 65) or Creamy Crab Dip (page 64)!

- Use leftover egg yolks to make Hollandaise Sauce (page 42) or Quick Béarnaise Sauce (page 23), or homemade mayo (page 20).

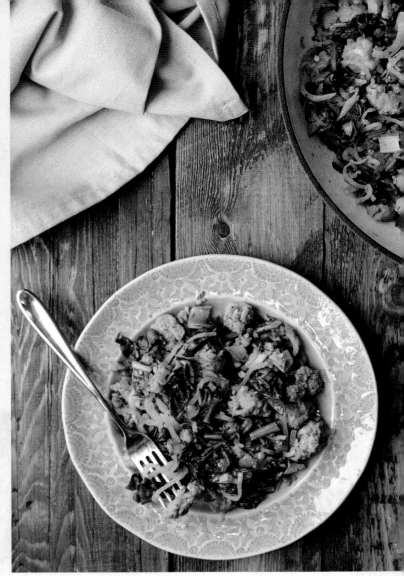

11) PLAN YOUR MEALS IN ADVANCE.

Proper planning means less wasting and bingeing. Planning is also key to a successful diet, which is why I focused on it when my partner and I created the KetoDiet App. I usually plan my meals every 5 to 7 days, and then prepare them 1 to 3 days ahead. Keep in mind that your plans may occasionally change—you might end up eating out, or may not be hungry—so always be prepared to make adjustments to your meal plan.

Always have keto-friendly foods on hand, even if you don't have time to cook. Boiled eggs, cheese (if you can eat dairy), non-starchy vegetables, avocados, cooked meat, responsibly sourced canned fish, and nuts and seeds (ideally soaked and dehydrated) will help you avoid bingeing.

Quick Keto Food List

Following a healthy, low-carb diet can seem challenging, especially if you're new to it. Here's a quick guide to keto-friendly foods that'll help you make the right choices. (To find a comprehensive ketogenic food list, check out my blog: www.ketodietapp.com/blog.)

EAT

Animal sources

• Organic or pastured eggs

• Grass-fed and wild animal sources: outdoor-reared pork, wild-caught fish, and grass-fed beef

• Organ meats: liver, kidneys, and heart

• Raw, full-fat dairy: yogurt, cheese, cream, and butter

Fats

• Use ghee, coconut oil, lard, duck fat, or tallow for high-heat cooking.

• Use extra-virgin olive oil, avocado oil, or macadamia nut oil for light cooking and salads.

• Other sources of healthy fats include nuts, seeds, nut and seed butters, coconut, avocado, and cacao butter. Beware of cashew nuts and pistachios: they're relatively high in carbs.

Fruits and vegetables

• Include non-starchy vegetables in your diet, such as leafy greens, cabbage, cauliflower, zucchini, broccoli, tomatoes, peppers, radishes, turnips, rutabaga, cucumber, celery, eggplant, asparagus, sea vegetables, onion, and garlic.

• Eat low-carb fruits such as berries, lemon, lime, rhubarb, coconut, and avocado.

When should you buy organic? Not all fruits and vegetables need to be labeled organic to be safe to eat. So which ones are worth paying for? Simple! If it's on the Dirty Dozen list (www.ewg.org), always buy organic.

Condiments, sweeteners, and packaged foods

• Herbs and spices (fresh or dried)

• Unsweetened tomato products, pumpkin purée, mustard, ketchup, beef stock, coconut aminos, fish sauce, sour pickles, sauerkraut, etc.

• Healthy, low-carb sweeteners, such as stevia, erythritol, Swerve, monk fruit extract, and inulin-based sweeteners

• Dark chocolate (with a minimum of 85% cacao content) and raw cacao powder

• Quality protein powder (without additives), gelatin, collagen, gluten-free baking powder, baking soda, cream of tartar, etc.

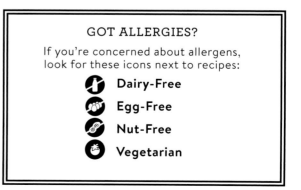

GOT ALLERGIES?

If you're concerned about allergens, look for these icons next to recipes:

Dairy-Free

Egg-Free

Nut-Free

Vegetarian

AVOID

- All grains and grain-based foods (bread, pasta, rice, crackers, pizza, oats, etc.)

- All foods high in carbs and sugar (cakes, cookies, ice cream, agave syrup, honey, tropical fruit and most high-sugar fruit, dried fruit, cocktails, beer, etc.)

- All processed, inflammatory fats (margarine, vegetable oil, canola oil, etc.) and processed products containing soy

- Products labeled "low-fat" and processed products labeled "low-carb"

- Condiments and foods that include carrageenan, MSG, sulphites, or artificial sweeteners

- Factory-farmed pork

- Farmed fish, fish high in mercury, and unsustainable fish

- Alcohol (Dry wine and spirits can be consumed in small amounts, but should be avoided for weight loss.)

EAT

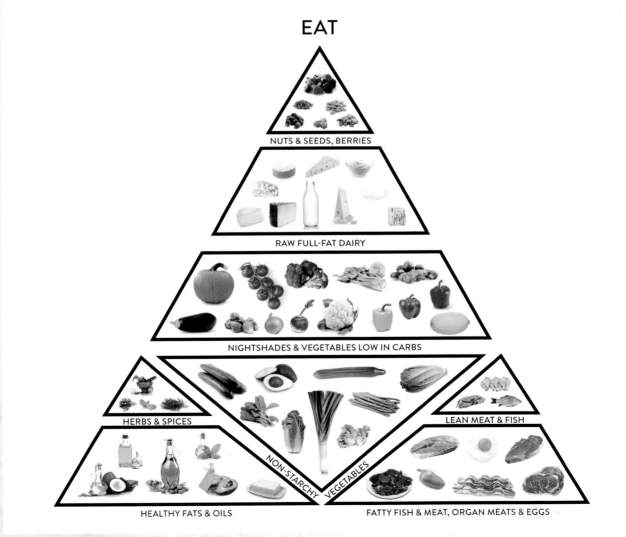

NUTS & SEEDS, BERRIES

RAW FULL-FAT DAIRY

NIGHTSHADES & VEGETABLES LOW IN CARBS

HERBS & SPICES

NON-STARCHY VEGETABLES

LEAN MEAT & FISH

HEALTHY FATS & OILS

FATTY FISH & MEAT, ORGAN MEATS & EGGS

AVOID

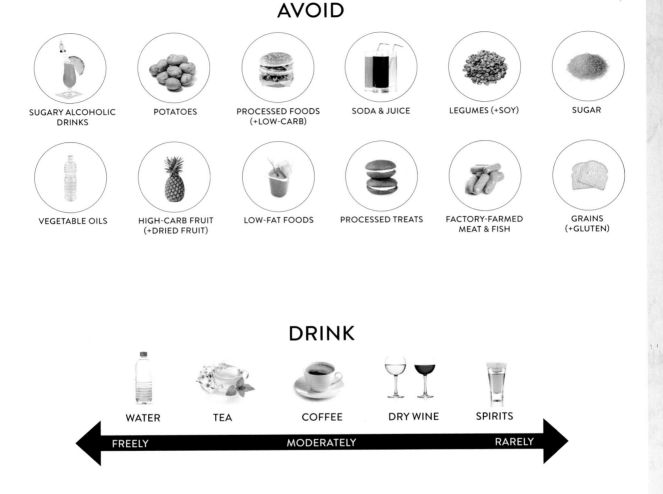

SUGARY ALCOHOLIC DRINKS	POTATOES	PROCESSED FOODS (+LOW-CARB)
SODA & JUICE	LEGUMES (+SOY)	SUGAR
VEGETABLE OILS	HIGH-CARB FRUIT (+DRIED FRUIT)	LOW-FAT FOODS
PROCESSED TREATS	FACTORY-FARMED MEAT & FISH	GRAINS (+GLUTEN)

DRINK

WATER · TEA · COFFEE · DRY WINE · SPIRITS

FREELY ← MODERATELY → RARELY

AN IMPORTANT NOTE ABOUT MEASUREMENTS

If you are following a ketogenic diet for specific health reasons, you should be aware that accuracy is vital in order for this diet to work. When measuring ingredients, always weigh them using a kitchen scale. Relying on cups or tablespoons can lead to inaccuracies that may affect the macronutrient composition of your meal. All it takes to shift your body out of ketosis is a few extra grams of carbohydrates. Plus, cups and tablespoons for dried products (flax meal, etc.) may vary depending on the brand.

CHAPTER 2:

The Basics

I rarely buy condiments because I want to have full control over what I eat. Most store-bought products contain sugar, preservatives, and other additives that are best avoided, so I make most of the ingredients I cook with myself. Don't worry: that's not as difficult as it sounds! In this chapter, you'll find recipes for everything from mayonnaise and pesto to gut-healing kimchi, sugar-free jam, and even homemade Mexican chorizo. A few recipes—like pork carnitas and kimchi—do take more than 30 minutes to prepare, but they require minimum hands-on time, so it's easy to multitask and to make a few of them at the same time.

Avocado and Kale Pesto

Making pesto at home is simple and it only takes a few minutes. This version is packed with healthy fats and electrolytes—especially potassium, which can help minimize the effects of "keto flu" during the first few weeks of keto-adaptation.

MAKES: 1½ CUPS (400 G/14.1 OZ) | HANDS-ON TIME: 5 MINUTES | OVERALL TIME: 5 MINUTES

1 medium (150 g/5.3 oz) avocado, peeled and seed removed

1 cup (35 g/1.2 oz) chopped kale or spinach

2 cups (30 g/1.1 oz) fresh basil leaves

4 cloves garlic, peeled

1 tablespoon (15 ml/0.5 oz) fresh lemon juice

½ cup (120 ml/4 oz) extra-virgin olive oil

1 teaspoon salt

¼ teaspoon black pepper

⅓ cup (45 g/1.6 oz) sunflower seeds or macadamia nuts

Optional: ⅓ cup (30 g/1.1 oz) grated Parmesan cheese

2 to 4 tablespoons (30 to 60 ml) extra-virgin olive oil

NUTRITION FACTS
PER SERVING
(2 TABLESPOONS/30 G/1.1 OZ)

Total carbs: 2.2 g | Fiber: 1.2 g
Net carbs: 1 g | Protein: 1.2 g
Fat: 11.6 g | Energy: 113 kcal
Macronutrient ratio: Calories from carbs (4%), protein (4%), fat (92%)

Place all the ingredients, except the 2 to 4 tablespoons (30 to 60 ml) of oil in a food processor or blender. Pulse until smooth. Transfer to a jar and pour 2 to 4 tablespoons of olive oil on top. Seal with a lid and refrigerate. You can keep your pesto in the fridge for up to 1 to 2 weeks. Whenever you use the pesto, always remember to add a thin layer of olive oil on top before you place it back in the fridge.

To preserve pesto for longer, spoon it into an ice cube tray and place in the freezer. Once frozen, empty the ice cube tray into a resealable plastic bag. Keep your frozen pesto cubes for up to 6 months.

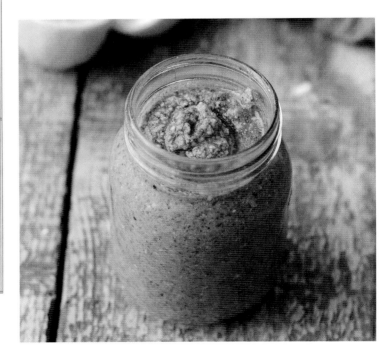

Mayonnaise

Mayonnaise is one of the most basic keto-friendly condiments. And, if you ferment it, it'll stay fresh for several months! Use the leftover egg whites to make Candied Spiced Cocoa Pecans (page 180).

MAKES: ABOUT 2 CUPS (480 G/16.9 OZ) | HANDS-ON TIME: 15 MINUTES | OVERALL TIME: 15 MINUTES

- 2 pastured egg yolks, at room temperature
- 2 teaspoons (10 g/0.2 oz) Dijon mustard
- 1½ cups (360 ml/12 fl oz) mild olive oil (or macadamia, avocado, or walnut oil)
- 2 tablespoons (30 ml/1 oz) fresh lemon juice
- 2 tablespoons (30 ml/1 oz) apple cider vinegar
- ½ teaspoon sea salt
- Optional: 2 tablespoons whey (30 ml/1 oz), or powder from 1 to 2 probiotic capsules

Place the yolks and Dijon mustard into a bowl, and mix until well combined. Using an electric mixer or hand whisk to mix as you go, drizzle in the oil very slowly. Start with just a few drops to make sure the mixture doesn't break.

Keep drizzling in the oil until the mixture starts to look more like the consistency of mayonnaise. Steadily pour in the oil until all of it is incorporated. Keep mixing until the mayo reaches the desired thickness. If it doesn't seem thick enough, add a bit more oil.

Mix in the lemon juice and vinegar—this will turn the mixture a light yellow color. Season with salt. If you think the consistency is too thick, add a few drops of water or lemon juice. Transfer the mayonnaise to a glass container and seal tightly. You can store it in the fridge for up to 1 week.

Optionally, mix in the whey and combine with the mayo. Transfer the mayonnaise to a jar, cover loosely with a lid or a cloth, and let it sit on a kitchen counter for 8 hours. This is essential in order to activate the enzymes that will keep your mayo fresh. After 8 hours, refrigerate and use within the next 3 months.

NUTRITION FACTS PER SERVING (1 TABLESPOON/15 G/0.5 OZ)

Total carbs: 0.1 g | Fiber: 0 g | Net carbs: 0.1 g | Protein: 0.2 g | Fat: 12.5 g | Energy: 111 kcal
Macronutrient ratio: Calories from carbs (0%), protein (1%), fat (99%)

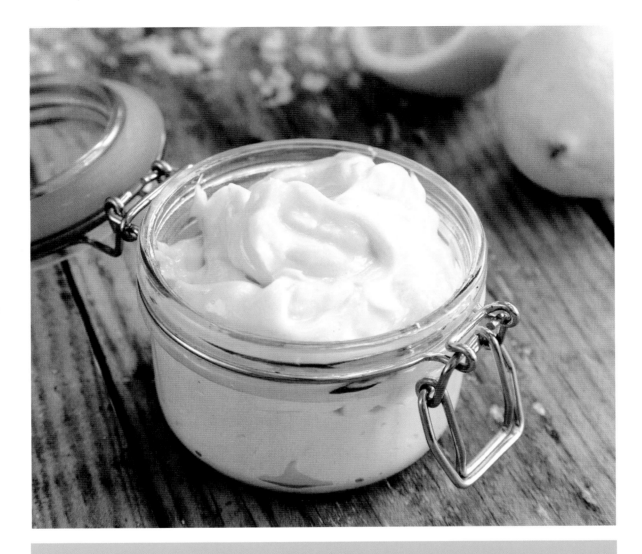

⌒ CONVERT YOUR MAYO INTO AIOLI OR TARTAR SAUCE IN A FEW EASY STEPS:

AIOLI: Add 2 to 4 cloves of minced garlic to the prepared mayonnaise.

TARTAR SAUCE: Mix ½ cup (110 g/3.9 oz) of the prepared mayonnaise with 2 small (50 g/1.8 oz) grated pickles, 2 tablespoons (30 ml/1 oz) lemon juice, ¼ teaspoon salt, and ⅛ teaspoon black pepper. Optionally, add 1 tablespoon (4 g/0.1 oz) of freshly chopped dill or parsley.

When using raw eggs, you should use only fresh, clean, properly refrigerated grade A or AA eggs with intact shells due to the slight risk of salmonella and other foodborne illnesses. Avoid contact between the yolks or whites and the outside of the shell. Prevent any risks by using eggs with pasteurized shells.

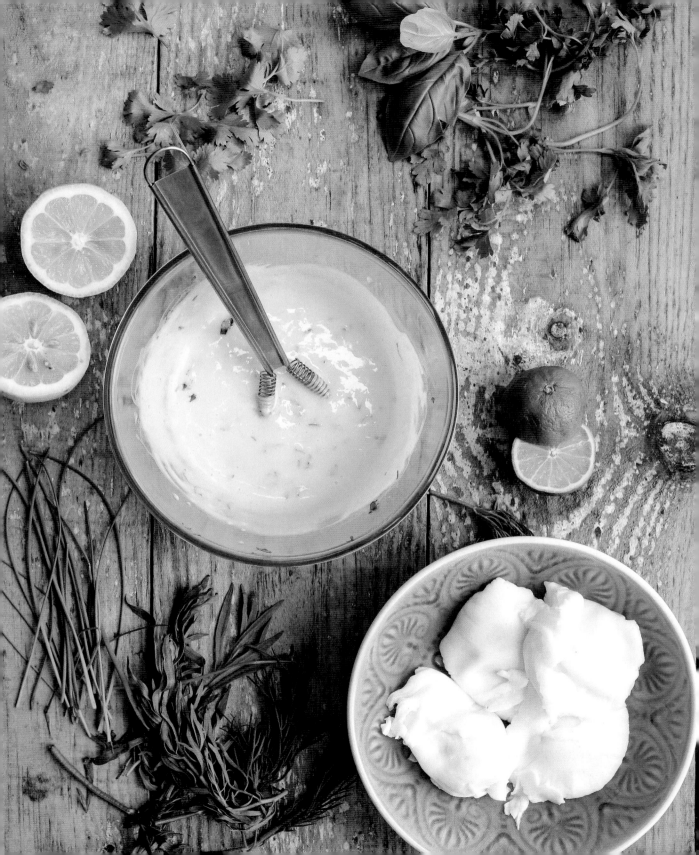

Quick Béarnaise Sauce

Béarnaise sauce is a high-fat condiment similar to hollandaise. It's perfect with steak, fish, and cooked vegetables, or simply poured over poached eggs.

MAKES: 2 SERVINGS (ABOUT ¼ CUP/60 ML/2 OZ) | HANDS-ON TIME: 15 MINUTES | OVERALL TIME: 15 MINUTES

¼ cup (60 g/2.1 oz) butter or ghee

3 tablespoons (15 g/0.5 oz) finely chopped shallot

1 tablespoon (4 g/0.1 oz) freshly chopped tarragon or other herbs of choice, divided

2 tablespoons (30 ml/1 oz) white wine vinegar

1 tablespoon (15 ml/0.5 oz) water

1 pastured egg yolk

1 tablespoon (15 ml/0.5 oz) fresh lemon or lime juice

¼ teaspoon Dijon mustard

Salt and pepper

Gently melt the butter and set aside; it should be warm, but not too hot. To make the béarnaise reduction, place the shallot, half of the chopped tarragon, vinegar, and water in a medium saucepan. Cook over low-medium heat for 2 to 3 minutes, until the liquid is reduced to just 1 to 2 tablespoons (15 to 30 ml/0.5 to 1 oz). Strain, discard the solids, and set aside until cool.

Fill a medium saucepan with a cup of water (235 ml/8 oz) and bring to a boil. Mix the egg yolk with the lemon juice and Dijon mustard in a heatproof bowl. Add the cooled vinegar mixture; place the bowl over the saucepan filled with water. The water should not touch the bottom of the bowl. Mix continuously until the sauce starts to thicken. Slowly pour the melted butter into the mixture until thick and creamy and stir constantly. If the sauce is too thick, add a splash of water.

Add the remaining tarragon, and season with salt and pepper. Serve immediately, or within 1 hour. Do not reheat or the sauce will separate. If you're only making it for yourself, halve this recipe and make a single serving.

⌐ To make this recipe dairy-free, use duck fat or lard instead of butter.

NUTRITION FACTS PER SERVING

Total carbs: 1.3 g | Fiber: 0.1 g | Net carbs: 1.1 g | Protein: 1.8 g | Fat: 26.7 g | Energy: 250 kcal
Macronutrient ratio: Calories from carbs (2%), protein (3%), fat (95%)

Kimchi

Fermented foods, including kimchi, are one of my favorite low-carb staples. Like sauerkraut, kimchi is made through a process called lacto-fermentation, which converts sugars into lactic acid. It's naturally low in carbs, and it's so good for your gut!

MAKES: 1 QUART JAR (950 ML) | HANDS-ON TIME: 30 MINUTES
OVERALL TIME (FERMENTATION): 3 TO 7 DAYS

Napa cabbage

1 to 2 tablespoons (17 to 34 g) salt

½ daikon radish (170 g/6 oz), julienned

4 medium (60 g/2.1 oz) spring onions, sliced

4 cloves garlic, minced

2 tablespoons (12 g/0.4 oz) finely chopped fresh ginger

¼ cup (28 g/1 oz) Korean hot pepper powder, or 2 tablespoons red pepper flakes

1 tablespoon (15 ml/0.5 oz) fish sauce or coconut aminos (for vegetarian kimchi)

Optional: 2 to 4 tablespoons erythritol or Swerve, or 5 to 10 drops liquid stevia extract

NUTRITION FACTS PER SERVING (½ CUP/70 G/2.5 OZ)

Total carbs: 2.5 g | Fiber: 1.2 g
Net carbs: 1.3 g | Protein: 1.3 g
Fat: 0 g | Energy: 19 kcal
Macronutrient ratio: Calories from carbs (50%), protein (50%), fat (0%)

Cut the cabbage lengthwise into quarters and remove the cores. Slice each quarter into 1-inch (2.5 cm) strips. Place the sliced cabbage into a large bowl and sprinkle with salt; start with 1 tablespoon (17 g/10.6 oz) and add more if needed. Using your hands, massage the salt into the cabbage. This will release the juices and soften the cabbage. Let the cabbage sit for 20 to 30 minutes.

Once the cabbage has softened, add the remaining ingredients. Mix until well combined. (Be sure to wear gloves when handling red pepper flakes.) Optionally, add the erythritol to balance out the spiciness of the chile powder.

Place the vegetables in a sterilized quart (950 ml) jar, pressing down until the brine rises above the vegetables. (If there isn't enough juice, add a little salted water until the vegetables are covered.) Leave at least 1 inch (2.5 cm) of space between the liquid and the top of the jar. Keep the vegetables under the brine by placing a small weighted jar on top. (This will prevent mold from forming on them.) Leave the jar in a warm spot in the kitchen to ferment for 3 to 7 days. The best way to tell whether the kimchi is ready is to taste it during the fermentation process; the longer you leave it, the stronger it'll taste. Once it's done, seal with a lid and store in the fridge for up to 6 months.

∽ To make this process easier, use a Fido jar. Simply place the vegetables in the Fido, leaving a small gap between the vegetables and the top of the jar, and close it. The advantage of a Fido jar is that you won't need to weight down the vegetables and worry about mold. The fermentation gases will escape through the rubber lid but no oxygen will get in. It's completely foolproof!

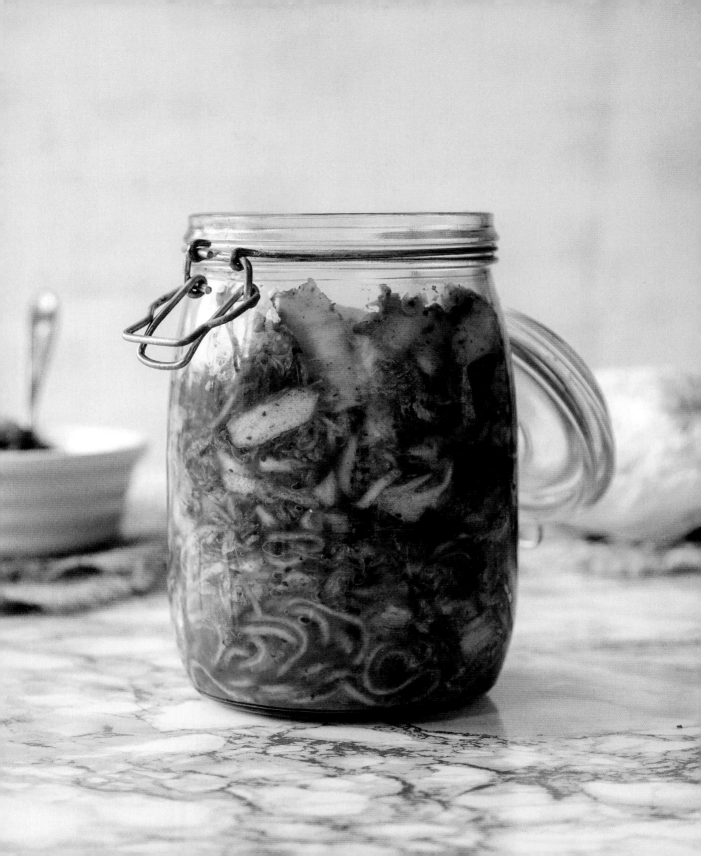

Mexican Chorizo

Making your own Mexican chorizo is easier than you think. Unlike Spanish chorizo, which is made from cured meat, Mexican chorizo is made with raw ground pork, and isn't always available in supermarkets. I use it for making breakfast patties, burgers, and quick one-pot meals.

MAKES: 2.5 POUNDS/1.15 KG | HANDS-ON TIME: 10 MINUTES
OVERALL TIME: 10 MINUTES + MARINATING

2.2 pounds (1 kg) ground fatty pork

6 tablespoons (36 g/1.3 oz) Mexican chile powder (ancho or guajillo)

1 tablespoon (3 g/0.1 oz) dried oregano, preferably Mexican

2 teaspoons (2 g/0.1 oz) ground cumin

1 teaspoon ground coriander

½ teaspoon ground cinnamon

½ teaspoon ground black pepper

¼ teaspoon ground allspice

¼ teaspoon cloves

2 teaspoons (11 g/0.4 oz) salt

4 bay leaves, crumbled

4 cloves garlic, minced

¼ cup (60 ml) white wine vinegar

Place all the ingredients in a bowl and mix until well combined (wear gloves if using your hands). Cover the bowl with plastic wrap and refrigerate for at least 2 hours—or ideally overnight—before using it in recipes. Store in the fridge for up to 3 days, or freeze in manageable portions for up to 3 months.

↶ If you can't find Mexican chile powder, you can use a combination of 5½ tablespoons (39 g/1.7 oz) of paprika and 1 to 2 teaspoons (2.6 to 5 g/0.1 to 0.2 oz) of red chile powder in place of 6 tablespoons (36 g/1.3 oz) of Mexican chile powder.

NUTRITION FACTS PER 3.5 OZ /100 G

Total carbs: 3 g | Fiber: 1.2 g | Net carbs: 1.8 g | Protein: 16 g | Fat: 19.7 g | Energy: 255 kcal
Macronutrient ratio: Calories from carbs (3%), protein (26%), fat (71%)

Pork Carnitas (a.k.a. Mexican Pulled Pork)

Pork carnitas is deliciously tender, slow-cooked meat that's crisped up
and flavored with orange, lime, and Mexican spices. I make it in advance for use in
salads and lettuce wraps, or I enjoy it on its own with a side of low-carb vegetables.

MAKES: 8 TO 10 SERVINGS | HANDS-ON TIME: 20 MINUTES | OVERALL TIME: 6 HOURS 20 MINUTES

2 teaspoons (2 g/0.1 oz) ground cumin

1 tablespoon (3 g/0.1 oz) dried oregano, preferably Mexican

1 tablespoon (17 g/0.6 oz) salt

1 teaspoon ground black pepper

4.4 pounds (2 kg) pork shoulder, bone in, or 3.5 pounds (1.6 kg) boneless pork shoulder

1 medium (110 g/3.9 oz) white onion, chopped

1 jalapeño pepper (14 g/0.5 oz), sliced, seeds and membranes removed

4 cloves garlic, minced

1 small (100 g/3.5 oz) orange, peeled and juiced

1 lime, juiced

¼ cup (60 ml) water

Optional: ¼ cup (55 g/1.9 oz) ghee or lard if using pork shoulder without under-skin fat layer

NUTRITION FACTS PER SERVING (ABOUT 5.3 OZ/ 150 G COOKED MEAT)

Total carbs: 4.4 g | Fiber: 1 g
Net carbs: 3.4 g | Protein: 34.9 g
Fat: 36.2 g | Energy: 490 kcal
Macronutrient ratio: Calories from carbs (3%), protein (29%), fat (68%)

Preheat your slow cooker to high. Combine the cumin, oregano, salt, and pepper in a small bowl. Rinse and dry the pork shoulder. Using a sharp knife, remove the skin and leave the fatty part on the pork shoulder (reserve the skin for making bone broth, page 13). Rub the prepared spices all over the pork shoulder and place it in a slow cooker with the onion, jalapeño, and garlic. Pour the orange and lime juices over the pork shoulder, and add the orange peel and water. Cover and cook for 6 hours.

When done, remove the meat from the slow cooker and set aside to cool slightly before shredding it into pieces with two forks. Discard the orange peel. Using a ladle, skim off the fat from the juices in the slow cooker and keep it aside in a bowl: you'll use the fat to fry your carnitas. Reserve the cooking juices in another bowl. If they come to more than 2 cups (475 ml/16 oz), pour them into a saucepan and cook until reduced.

Heat a pan greased with some of the reserved fat (alternatively, use ghee or lard). Place the shredded pork into the pan and press down. Cook for a few minutes until crisped up, and place on a serving plate. Pour over some of the cooking juices and serve. You can store the meat in the fridge for up to 5 days and reheat in a pan or in the oven as needed. To freeze, store in manageable batches for up to 6 months.

◌ Instead of a slow cooker, you can use a pressure cooker. Add about 1 cup (235 ml/8 oz) water and cook on high pressure for 45 to 50 minutes.

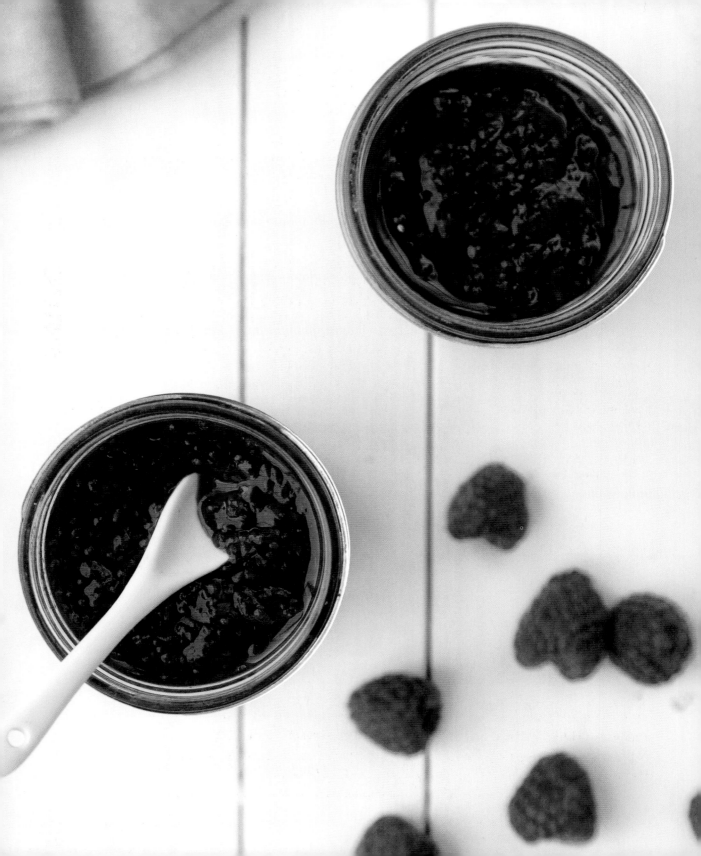

Raspberry Chia Jam

Making fruity, healthy berry jam couldn't be simpler.
You won't need to use any pectin. It's also super-nutritious, thanks to the
healthy fiber, protein, and omega-3 fatty acids in the chia seeds.

MAKES: 1¾ CUPS (455 G/16 OZ) | HANDS-ON TIME: 10 MINUTES | OVERALL TIME: 30 MINUTES

3 cups (370 g/13 oz) fresh or frozen raspberries

3 tablespoons (45 ml/1.5 oz) water

3 tablespoons (30 g/1.1 oz) erythritol or Swerve, or 10 to 15 drops liquid stevia extract

½ teaspoon vanilla bean powder or 1 to 2 teaspoons sugar-free vanilla extract

3 tablespoons (24 g/0.8 oz) chia seeds

Mash the raspberries using a fork or a blender. Place the crushed raspberries into a saucepan and add the water. Bring to a boil over medium heat and cook for 2 to 3 minutes to soften, then remove from the heat. Add the erythritol (or stevia) and vanilla powder. Mix well. Finally, add the chia seeds. Stir and let the mixture sit for at least 20 minutes to thicken and cool. Store in the fridge in a jar or an airtight container for up to 1 week.

⌐ To make the jam last longer, spoon it into an ice cube tray and freeze. Once frozen, place the berry ice cubes in a freezer bag and store in the freezer for up to 6 months.

NUTRITION FACTS PER SERVING (2 TABLESPOONS/40 G/1.4 OZ)

Total carbs: 4.9 g | Fiber: 2.9 g | Net carbs: 2 g | Protein: 0.8 g | Fat: 0.9 g | Energy: 29 kcal
Macronutrient ratio: Calories from carbs (42%), protein (17%), fat (41%)

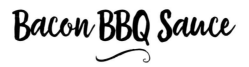

Bacon BBQ Sauce

Ditch that bottled barbecue sauce; it's full of sugar and additives.
Instead, make your own in just a few easy steps. This sweet-and-spicy sauce
adds fantastic flavor to just about any type of meat—and to grilled vegetables, too.

MAKES: 2½ CUPS (600 G/1.3 LB) | HANDS-ON TIME: 20 TO 25 MINUTES | OVERALL TIME: 20 TO 25 MINUTES

1 tablespoon (15 g/0.5 oz) ghee or lard

4 large slices (120 g/4.2 oz) bacon, chopped

1 small (70 g/2.5 oz) white onion, chopped, or 2 teaspoons (2 g/0.07 oz) onion powder

4 cloves garlic, minced, or 1 teaspoon garlic powder

1 small can (200 g/7.1 oz) chopped tomatoes, unsweetened

½ cup (100 g/3.5 oz) pumpkin purée, unsweetened

¼ cup (60 g/2.1 oz) tomato paste, unsweetened

¼ cup (60 ml) chicken stock, vegetable stock, or bone broth (page 13)

¼ cup (60 ml) apple cider vinegar

2 tablespoons (30 ml/1 oz) coconut aminos

2 tablespoons (20 g/0.7 oz) erythritol or Swerve, or 5 to 10 drops liquid stevia extract

½ to 1 teaspoon chili powder

⅛ teaspoon ground allspice

⅛ teaspoon ground cloves

½ teaspoon salt, preferably smoked

¼ teaspoon ground black pepper

Heat a large saucepan or Dutch oven greased with ghee. Add the chopped bacon. Cook over a medium-low heat until lightly browned. Add the onion and garlic, and cook for 3 to 5 minutes. Add all the remaining ingredients. Cook for 10 to 15 minutes, or until the desired thickness is reached. Transfer to a blender and pulse until smooth (or chunky, if you like). Once cool, store in the fridge in a jar or an airtight container for up to 1 month. To keep it fresh for longer, spoon it into an ice cube tray and freeze. Once frozen, place the ice cubes in a freezer bag and store in the freezer for up to 6 months.

NUTRITION FACTS PER SERVING (1 TABLESPOON/15 G/0.5 OZ)

Total carbs: 0.9 g | Fiber: 0.2 g | Net carbs: 0.7 g | Protein: 0.6 g | Fat: 0.8 g | Energy: 13 kcal
Macronutrient ratio: Calories from carbs (23%), protein (19%), fat (58%)

Pico De Gallo (Fresh Tomato Salsa)

When tomatoes are in season, I make a batch of fresh tomato salsa
almost every other day. It's perfect as a condiment, as a side with grilled meat,
with my Taco Frittata (page 74), or with my Beef Fajitas (page 140).
I like my salsa on the spicy side, but feel free to adjust the heat to taste.

MAKES: 3 CUPS (750 G/1.7 LB) | HANDS-ON TIME: 10 MINUTES | OVERALL TIME: 10 MINUTES

2 to 3 medium (28 g/1 oz) jalapeño or
serrano peppers

1 small (75 g/2.6 oz) red bell pepper

1 pound (450 g) tomatoes

1 small (70 g/2.5 oz) white or red
onion

4 cloves garlic, minced

2 medium (30 g/1.1 oz) spring onions,
sliced

2 tablespoons (30 ml/1 oz) lime juice

¼ cup (60 ml) extra-virgin olive oil

½ cup (10 g/0.4 oz) loosely packed
fresh cilantro, chopped

½ teaspoon ground cumin

½ teaspoon salt, or to taste

¼ teaspoon ground black pepper

Halve the jalapeño and bell peppers, and remove the seeds
and membranes. Finely dice the peppers, tomatoes, and
onion, and place in a mixing bowl. Add the garlic, spring
onions, lime juice, olive oil, cilantro, cumin, salt, and
pepper. Mix well until combined and serve, or transfer to a
jar with a lid and seal. Refrigerate and store for up to 3 days.

**NUTRITION FACTS PER
¼ CUP/60 ML**

Total carbs: 3.2 g | Fiber: 0.9 g
Net carbs: 2.3 g | Protein: 0.6 g
Fat: 4.6 g | Energy: 55 kcal
Macronutrient ratio: Calories from
carbs (17%), protein (5%), fat (78%)

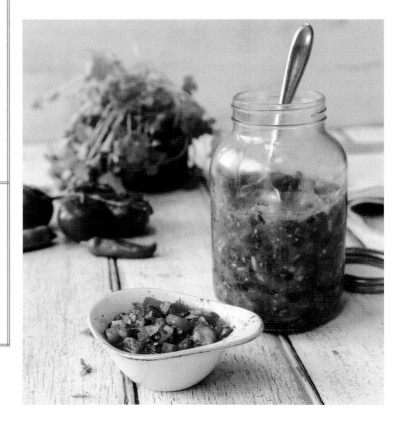

CHAPTER 3

Breakfast

For decades we've been eating cereal, porridge, and toast for breakfast—the seemingly healthy options dictated by the food industry. Before I started eating low-carb, I used to have a bowl of cereal with dried fruit and low-fat milk for breakfast almost every day. After all, morning is when our bodies need extra carbs, right? Well, that didn't work for me. I felt tired and low-energy all morning, and I often reached for even more "healthy" energy bars to keep me going—which made me feel even worse.

   When I switched to a low-carb approach, things improved dramatically. The reason is simple: When you wake up in the morning, your body is in fat-burning mode. A low-carb meal will keep you fuller for longer, help you to control cravings, and will keep your energy levels steady all day. So, be sure to keep your carb intake low in the morning, and consume the majority of your carbs later in the day. To that end, this chapter features my favorite quick-prep, high-fat, breakfast meals such as hash, meat patties, egg dishes, pancakes, and even keto-friendly cereal. Get ready to become a morning person!

Greek Breakfast Hash

Greeks have remarkably long life spans, and one of the reasons is that they use extra-virgin olive oil every day. This recipe features some of the best low-carb Greek staples: eggplant, Halloumi cheese, and heart-healthy extra-virgin olive oil.

MAKES: 2 SERVINGS | HANDS-ON TIME: 15 MINUTES | OVERALL TIME: 25 MINUTES

1 medium (250 g/8.8 oz) eggplant

1 package (125 g/4.4 oz) Halloumi

1 clove garlic, peeled and finely chopped

2 tablespoons (30 g/1.1 oz) ghee or lard

1 teaspoon dried oregano

2 tablespoons (30 ml/1 oz) extra-virgin olive oil

1 teaspoon balsamic vinegar

Optional: 2 to 4 large pastured eggs

Roughly dice the eggplant and the Halloumi into 1-inch (2 cm) pieces. Cook the garlic in a large pan greased with ghee over medium heat for 1 minute, until fragrant. Add the Halloumi and cook for 5 to 8 minutes, until browned on both sides. Add the diced eggplant and oregano, and cook for another 5 minutes. Stir, cover, and cook for 5 more minutes, or until the eggplant is soft. Remove from the heat and set aside.

Mix the olive oil and balsamic vinegar in a small bowl. Place the cooked eggplant and Halloumi hash on serving plates. Drizzle with the olive oil and balsamic vinegar mixture. Optionally, serve with fried eggs (page 10).

NUTRITION FACTS PER SERVING

Total carbs: 10.2 g | Fiber: 4.2 g
Net carbs: 6 g | Protein: 13.9 g
Fat: 45.7 g | Energy: 500 kcal
Macronutrient ratio: Calories from carbs (5%), protein (11%), fat (84%)

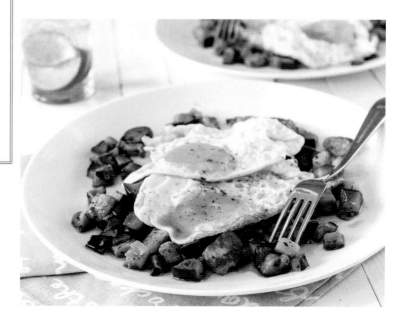

Cheesy Grain-Free Waffles

These keto-friendly waffles are so versatile! I serve them as a side dish with Mexican Pulled Pork (page 27), soups, and all sorts of salads. They also make a fantastic alternative to English muffins if you're making eggs Benedict.

MAKES: 2 SERVINGS (4 WAFFLES) | HANDS-ON TIME: 15 MINUTES | OVERALL TIME: 15 MINUTES

3 large pastured eggs

¼ cup (60 g/2.1 oz) cream cheese, at room temperature

⅓ cup (30 g/1.1 oz) grated Parmesan cheese

½ cup (56 g/2 oz) grated Cheddar cheese

3 tablespoons (21 g/0.7 oz) flax meal, or 4 tablespoons (24 g/0.8 oz) almond flour

1 tablespoon (8 g/0.3 oz) coconut flour

1 teaspoon mixed dried Italian herbs (basil, oregano, thyme)

½ teaspoon garlic powder

½ teaspoon onion powder

½ teaspoon gluten-free baking powder

Salt and pepper

Optional: serve with poached or fried eggs (page 10), and Hollandaise Sauce (page 42) or Quick Béarnaise Sauce (page 23)

Place the eggs and cream cheese in a large bowl. Mix well. Add the Parmesan and Cheddar, plus all the dry ingredients, and mix well. Pour the batter into a preheated waffle maker, close, and cook for 1 to 2 minutes, or until crisped up and cooked through. When done, transfer to a plate and let the waffles cool for a few minutes before serving.

Store any leftover waffles in an airtight container in the fridge for up to 5 days, or freeze for up to 3 months. They're especially delicious when topped with poached eggs and Hollandaise Sauce.

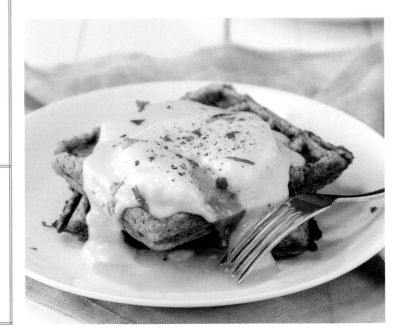

NUTRITION FACTS PER SERVING (2 WAFFLES)

Total carbs: 8.2 g | Fiber: 4 g
Net carbs: 4.2 g | Protein: 26.8 g
Fat: 33.8 g | Energy: 431 kcal
Macronutrient ratio: Calories from carbs (4%), protein (25%), fat (71%)

Breakfast Sausage Patties

This is the ultimate make-ahead meal, and it's so versatile that you can enjoy it any time of day. I always make these Breakfast Sausage Patties in batches for freezing, and I reheat them as needed. They're great with eggs, spinach/chard, cheese, and avocado.

MAKES: 4 SERVINGS (12 PATTIES) | HANDS-ON TIME: 10 MINUTES | OVERALL TIME: 20 MINUTES

1.1 pounds (500 g) ground pork

1 large pastured egg

2 cloves garlic, minced

½ teaspoon dried sage

½ teaspoon dried thyme

¼ teaspoon fennel seeds

⅛ teaspoon ground nutmeg

⅛ teaspoon ground cloves

½ teaspoon salt

Pinch of black pepper

2 tablespoons (30 g/1.1 oz) ghee or lard for frying

Place the ground pork, egg, garlic, sage, thyme, fennel, nutmeg, cloves, salt, and pepper into a bowl, and combine.

Using your hands, form the mixture into 12 small patties. Grease a large pan with ghee and heat over medium-high heat. Fry the patties in batches for 4 to 5 minutes per side. (Don't flip them too early or they'll get stuck on the pan.)

Season with salt and pepper to taste, and eat immediately with fried eggs, sliced avocado, or braised spinach. Or, once the patties cool down, store them in the fridge for up to 5 days or freeze for up to 3 months.

NUTRITION FACTS PER SERVING (3 PATTIES)

Total carbs: 1.8 g | Fiber: 0.4 g
Net carbs: 1.4 g | Protein: 24.3 g
Fat: 28.9 g | Energy: 364 kcal
Macronutrient ratio: Calories from carbs (1%), protein (27%), fat (72%)

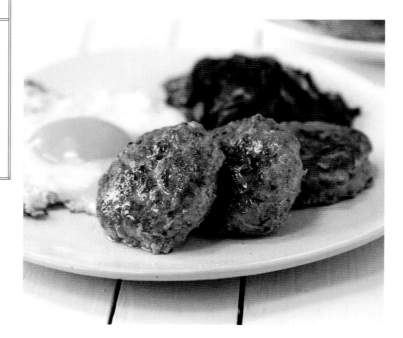

Middle Eastern Hash

This is my favorite "anytime" meal because it's quick and tastes fantastic. It's great as a filling breakfast or brunch, but it makes a light, healthy, flavorful lunch or dinner, too.

MAKES: 2 SERVINGS | HANDS-ON TIME: 20 MINUTES | OVERALL TIME: 20 MINUTES

2 tablespoons (30 g/1.1 oz) ghee, lard, or virgin coconut oil

1 small (70 g/2.5 oz) white or yellow onion, diced

1 clove garlic, minced

½ medium (60 g/2.1 oz) green pepper, sliced

½ medium (60 g/2.1 oz) red pepper, sliced

1 medium (100 g/3.5 oz) tomato, roughly chopped

½ teaspoon ground cumin

½ teaspoon paprika

⅛ teaspoon chili powder

2 tablespoons (8 g/0.3 oz) freshly chopped cilantro or parsley, plus more for garnish

Salt and pepper

1 small bunch (100 g/3.5 oz) kale, chopped, stems removed

¼ cup (60 ml/2 oz) chicken stock, bone broth, or vegetable stock (page 13)

4 large pastured eggs

1 tablespoon (15 ml/0.5 oz) fresh lemon juice

2 tablespoons (30 ml/1 oz) extra-virgin olive oil

Heat a large pan or pot greased with ghee. (It should be deep enough to fit all the vegetables.) Once hot, add the onion and cook over medium-high heat until fragrant, about 3 minutes. Add the garlic and peppers, and cook for 2 to 3 minutes more, stirring occasionally. Add the tomato and all the spices and seasonings and mix well. Add the kale and chicken stock, mix, and cook for a few minutes until the kale is tender, 5 to 7 minutes.

Use a spatula to make 4 wells in the mixture. Crack 1 egg into each well and cook until the whites are opaque and cooked through and the egg yolks are still runny. Remove from the heat, drizzle the hash with the lemon juice and olive oil, and garnish with more cilantro.

To speed things up, you can use whole chard leaves (including stalks) or collard greens: Swiss chard takes just a minute to cook, while kale takes 5 to 7 minutes.

NUTRITION FACTS PER SERVING

Total carbs: 12.2 g | Fiber: 3.6 g | Net carbs: 8.6 g | Protein: 15.7 g | Fat: 39.2 g | Energy: 460 kcal
Macronutrient ratio: Calories from carbs (8%), protein (14%), fat (78%)

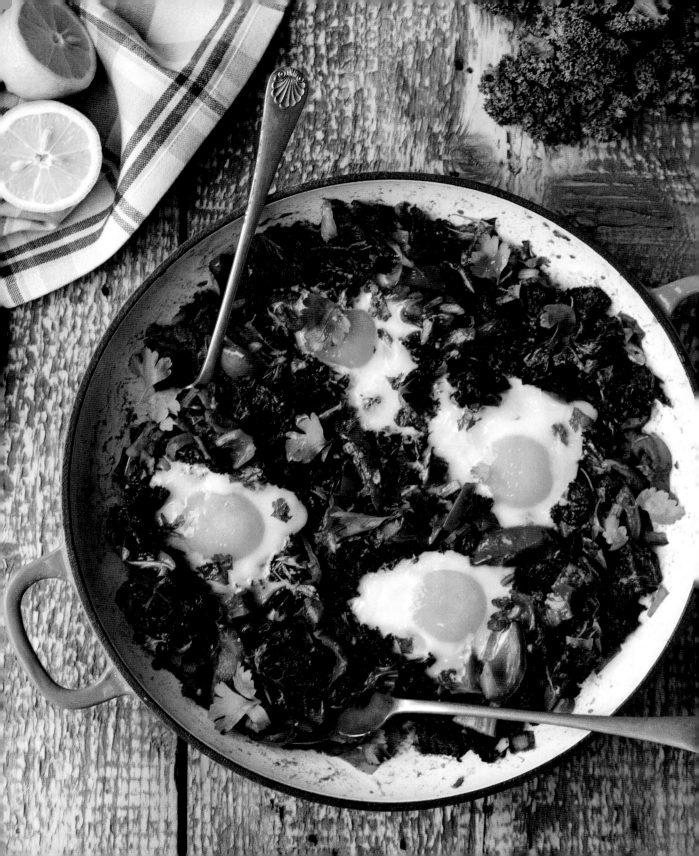

Sausage and Turnip Hash

This hearty low-carb hash is especially lovely on cool fall mornings. Serve it on its own, or alongside fried eggs (page 10). When you're buying pork—including sausage meat—always opt for organic. Factory-farmed animals live in terrible conditions, and they're fed with antibiotics that make their way onto your plate.

MAKES: 4 SERVINGS | HANDS-ON TIME: 15 MINUTES | OVERALL TIME: 25 MINUTES

1 pound (450 g) gluten-free sausage meat

2 tablespoons (30 g/1.1 oz) ghee or lard, divided

1 small (70 g/2.5 oz) white or yellow onion, finely chopped

2 cloves garlic, minced

1 medium (200 g/7.1 oz) turnip, peeled and diced into ½-inch (1 cm) pieces

½ teaspoon dried herbs (marjoram, rosemary, or thyme)

¼ cup (60 ml/2 oz) chicken stock or bone broth (page 13)

7.1 ounces (200 g) Swiss chard, roughly chopped (remove stalks and chop them separately)

Salt and pepper

Place the sausage meat in a large pan greased with 1 tablespoon (15 g/0.5 oz) of the ghee and cook over medium-high heat until browned on all sides, 8 to 10 minutes. Use a slotted spoon to transfer the meat to a bowl.

Grease the pan in which you cooked the sausage with the remaining 1 tablespoon (15 g/0.5 oz) ghee. Add the onion and garlic. Cook over medium-high heat until fragrant, 3 minutes. Add the turnip, dried herbs, and chicken stock, and cook over medium-low heat for 10 minutes, stirring occasionally.

When the turnip is tender yet still crisp, add the chard stalks, and cook for another 1 to 2 minutes. Finally, add the chard leaves, stir, and cook for 1 minute. Place the cooked sausage back into the pan, mix, and season the hash with salt and pepper to taste. Serve immediately.

NUTRITION FACTS PER SERVING

Total carbs: 7.9 g | Fiber: 2.2 g | Net carbs: 5.7 g | Protein: 17.9 g | Fat: 43.2 g | Energy: 493 kcal
Macronutrient ratio: Calories from carbs (5%), protein (15%), fat (80%)

Easy Cauliflower and Egg Hash

I grew up in a village where my parents kept a big garden. They grew their own fruit and vegetables, and they kept their own chickens—and they still do! My mother used to make this Easy Cauliflower and Egg Hash almost every week. You'll be surprised at how well eggs and cauliflower work together. Plus, it's one of the simplest meals imaginable.

MAKES: 4 SERVINGS | HANDS-ON TIME: 15 MINUTES | OVERALL TIME: 25 MINUTES

1 medium (500 g/1.1 lb) head cauliflower, cut into florets

6 large pastured eggs

Salt and pepper

¼ cup (55 g/1.9 oz) ghee or lard

1 small (70 g/2.5 oz) white or yellow onion, chopped

¼ teaspoon ground caraway, or ½ teaspoon whole caraway seeds

2 tablespoons (6 g/0.2 oz) chopped chives or spring onion

Optional: Crispy bacon slices

Place the cauliflower florets in a steamer and cook for 8 to 10 minutes, until tender. Remove from the heat, take off the lid, and let the florets cool. Cut the florets into 1-inch (2.5 cm) pieces. Set aside.

Crack the eggs into a bowl, and add salt and pepper to taste. Whisk with a fork and set aside. Grease a large pan with the ghee and heat over medium heat. Once hot, add the onion, and cook until fragrant and lightly browned.

Add the chopped cauliflower and caraway, and cook for 1 to 2 minutes. Add the whisked eggs and continue to mix with a spatula until the eggs are cooked. Remove from the heat and top with the chives. Optionally, serve with crispy bacon slices.

NUTRITION FACTS PER SERVING

Total carbs: 8.4 g | Fiber: 3 g | Net carbs: 5.4 g | Protein: 12.1 g | Fat: 21.3 g | Energy: 270 kcal
Macronutrient ratio: Calories from carbs (8%), protein (19%), fat (73%)

Mexican Hash

Prepare this Mexican hash the night before and just reheat it in the morning—or whenever you're hungry! It goes with just about anything, but I like to top mine with eggs or sliced avocado.

MAKES: 4 SERVINGS | HANDS-ON TIME: 15 MINUTES | OVERALL TIME: 25 MINUTES

8.8 ounces (250 g) Mexican Chorizo (Make your own! See page 26)

2 tablespoons (30 g/1.1 oz) ghee or lard, divided

2 cups (230 g/8.1 oz) diced pumpkin (½-inch [1 cm] pieces)

1 medium bunch (200 g/7.1 oz) kale or Swiss chard

Place the chorizo in a large pan greased with 1 tablespoon (15 g/0.5 oz) of the ghee and cook until browned on all sides, 8 to 10 minutes. Use a slotted spoon to transfer to a bowl.

Add the remaining 1 tablespoon (15 g/0.5 oz) ghee and diced pumpkin to the pan. Cook over medium heat for 6 to 8 minutes, stirring occasionally. Add the kale, cover, and cook for 5 to 7 minutes, until soft and wilted but still green. (If you're using Swiss chard instead of kale, cook for just 1 to 2 minutes.) Place the cooked chorizo back into the pan to reheat for 1 minute, and serve.

∽ Optionally, serve with sliced avocado, poached or fried eggs (page 10), and Quick Béarnaise (page 23) or Hollandaise Sauce (page 42). To give your hollandaise a Mexican kick, use lime juice instead of lemon juice, and add a pinch of cayenne pepper and some fresh cilantro.

∽ Can't get fresh pumpkin? Try sweet potato instead. Just keep in mind that sweet potato contains three times more carbs than pumpkin and should be used sparingly.

NUTRITION FACTS PER SERVING

Total carbs: 8.4 g | Fiber: 2 g | Net carbs: 6.4 g | Protein: 11.5 g | Fat: 20.1 g | Energy: 256 kcal
Macronutrient ratio: Calories from carbs (7%), protein (18%), fat (76%)

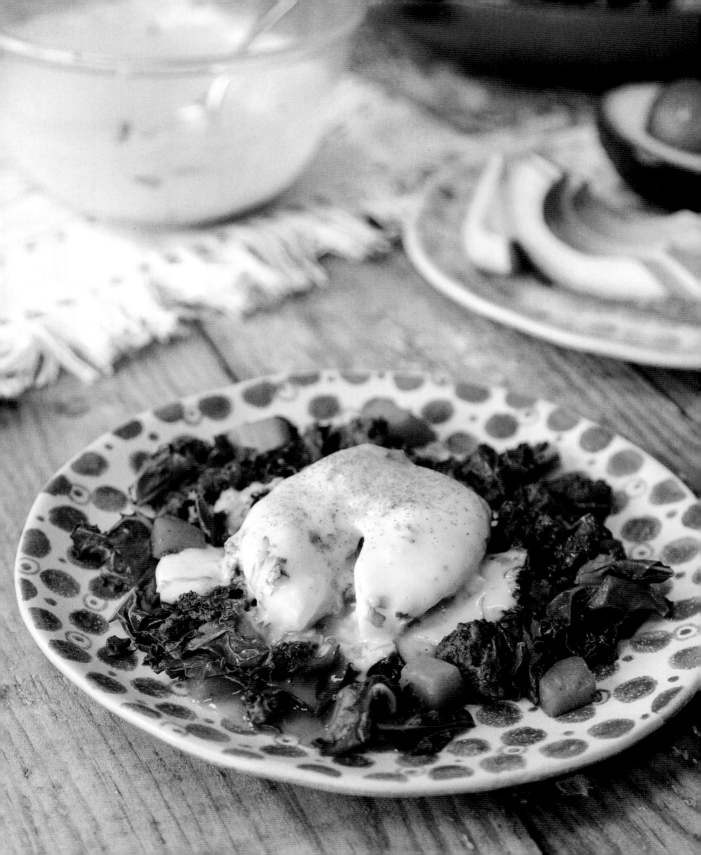

Eggs Royale Two Ways

This breakfast classic is one of the easiest ways to prepare eggs. You can use all sorts of low-carb vegetables to make this dish, but nutrient-rich broccoli and asparagus are my top picks.

MAKES: 2 SERVINGS | HANDS-ON TIME: 20 MINUTES | OVERALL TIME: 20 MINUTES

HOLLANDAISE SAUCE:

¼ cup (60 g/2.1 oz) butter or ghee

2 pastured egg yolks

2 tablespoons (30 ml/1 oz) fresh lemon juice

1 to 2 tablespoons (15 to 30 ml/0.5 to 1 oz) water

½ teaspoon Dijon mustard

EGGS ROYALE:

2 large pastured eggs

8.5 ounces (240 g) broccolini or asparagus

Salt and pepper

Fresh herbs, such as chives, for garnish

To make the hollandaise sauce, gently melt the butter and set aside; it should be warm, but not too hot. Fill a medium saucepan with a cup of water and bring to a boil. In a separate bowl, mix the egg yolks with the lemon juice, water, and Dijon mustard. (Use the leftover egg whites to make Candied Spiced Cocoa Pecans on page 180.)

Place the bowl over the saucepan filled with water. The water should not touch the bottom of the bowl. Keep mixing until the sauce starts to thicken. Slowly pour the melted butter into the mixture until thick and creamy, and stir constantly. If the sauce is too thick, add a splash of water. Set aside while you cook the eggs and vegetables.

To make the eggs royale, poach the eggs following the instructions on page 10. Set aside and cook the vegetables. Bring a saucepan filled with salted water to boil. Add the broccoli (or asparagus) and cook for 3 to 4 minutes until crisp-tender (1 to 2 minutes for asparagus). Drain and keep warm.

Divide the cooked broccoli (or asparagus) between two serving plates, add a poached egg to each, and top with the hollandaise sauce. Season with salt and pepper to taste and garnish with fresh herbs.

⌒ Hollandaise should be served immediately, or within 1 hour. Do not reheat or the sauce will separate. If you only make it for yourself, halve this recipe, and prepare one serving at a time.

NUTRITION FACTS PER SERVING

(BROCCOLINI) Total carbs: 9.9 g | Fiber: 3.2 g | Net carbs: 6.7 g | Protein: 12.7 g | Fat: 34.2 g | Energy: 387 kcal
Macronutrient ratio: Calories from carbs (7%), protein (13%), fat (80%)

(ASPARAGUS) Total carbs: 6.6 g | Fiber: 2.6 g | Net carbs: 4 g | Protein: 12 g | Fat: 33.9 g | Energy: 370 kcal
Macronutrient ratio: Calories from carbs (4%), protein (13%), fat (83%)

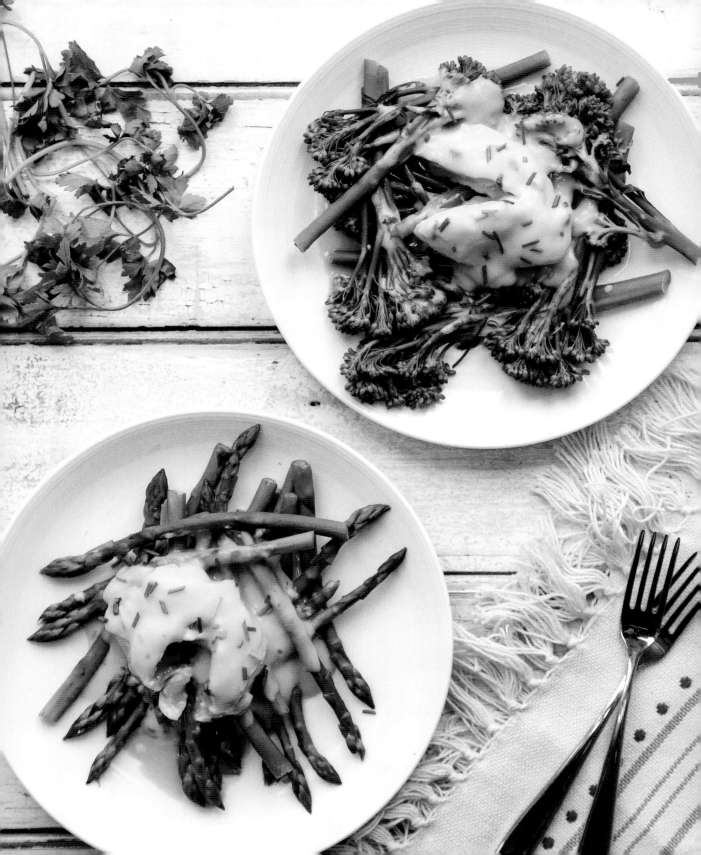

Good-for-Your-Gut Scrambles

Scrambled eggs with gut-healing kimchi have become a breakfast staple in my house. Eggs are high in B vitamins, choline, and the best-quality protein—and that means you'll feel fuller for longer.

MAKES: 2 SERVINGS | HANDS-ON TIME: 5 MINUTES | OVERALL TIME: 10 MINUTES

6 large pastured eggs

2 tablespoons (30 g/1.1 oz) ghee, lard, or virgin coconut oil

1 cup (70 g/2.5 oz) sliced shiitake or brown mushrooms

1 cup (70 g/2.5 oz) chopped leafy greens, such as bok choy, chard, or spinach

1 cup (140 g/5 oz) Kimchi (Make your own! See page 24)

Salt and pepper

Crack the eggs into a bowl and whisk with a fork. Grease a large pan with the ghee and heat over medium heat. Add the mushrooms and cook for 4 to 5 minutes. Add the greens and cook for 1 to 2 minutes. Add the kimchi and eggs, and cook until the eggs turn opaque, 2 to 3 minutes. Season with salt and pepper to taste.

If you love mushrooms, add some reserved mushroom stems from Eggs Florentine in Portobello Mushrooms (page 45). Also, you can use firm greens like kale here, but they take longer to cook. If using, add them to the pan together with the mushrooms and cook for 5 to 7 minutes before adding the kimchi.

NUTRITION FACTS PER SERVING

Total carbs: 6.8 g | Fiber: 2.5 g | Net carbs: 4.3 g | Protein: 21.4 g | Fat: 29.5 g | Energy: 386 kcal
Macronutrient ratio: Calories from carbs (5%), protein (23%), fat (72%)

Eggs Florentine in Portobello Mushrooms

Traditional eggs Florentine is made with poached eggs, spinach, and hollandaise sauce. This version is even more nutritious and filling, thanks to the addition of portobello mushrooms and omega-3-rich smoked salmon. It's sure to keep you satisfied until lunch.

MAKES: 2 SERVINGS | HANDS-ON TIME: 20 MINUTES | OVERALL TIME: 25 MINUTES

2 portobello mushrooms (150 g/5.3 oz)

Salt and pepper

1 tablespoon (15 g/0.5 oz) ghee or lard

2 large pastured eggs

7.1 ounces (200 g) spinach, fresh or cooked

3.5 ounces (100 g) smoked salmon

1 recipe Hollandaise Sauce (page 42)

Clean the mushrooms with a damp paper towel. Remove the stems and reserve for another recipe (like Good-for-Your-Gut Scrambles, page 44). Season the mushrooms with salt and pepper, and place on a hot pan greased with ghee, bottom-side up. Cook for 1 to 2 minutes, flip them over, and cover the pan. Cook for an additional 5 to 7 minutes, or until tender. Remove from the heat and set aside.

Prepare the poached eggs (page 10) and cook the spinach. To prepare fresh spinach, place it in a large pan and cook over medium heat for 1 to 2 minutes or until wilted, tossing gently with tongs. (If all the spinach doesn't fit into the pan at once, add more spinach to the pan in batches as it cooks down.) Remove from the pan and set aside.

To serve, place one mushroom, bottom-side up, on each serving plate. Top each with half the wilted spinach (squeeze out any excess water, if necessary), half the smoked salmon, and one poached egg. Finally, top with hollandaise sauce and serve immediately.

NUTRITION FACTS PER SERVING

Total carbs: 8.4 g | Fiber: 3.2 g | Net carbs: 5.2 g | Protein: 22.9 g | Fat: 44.1 g | Energy: 512 kcal
Macronutrient ratio: Calories from carbs (4%), protein (18%), fat (78%)

Full English Breakfast

Here, the traditional English breakfast gets a healthy, low-carb makeover. This recipe was inspired by the restaurant my partner and I visit for a full English breakfast every Sunday. The staff always makes us a special keto-friendly version, with extra avocado and spinach instead of toast or beans.

MAKES: 2 SERVINGS | HANDS-ON TIME: 15 MINUTES | OVERALL TIME: 20 MINUTES

2 large pastured eggs

2 tablespoons (30 g/1.1 oz) ghee, lard, or bacon grease

2 medium (100 g/3.5 oz) gluten-free sausages

2 large (60 g/2.1 oz) slices pastured bacon

2 cups (140 g/5 oz) sliced white mushrooms

Salt and pepper

7.1 ounces (200 g) cooked spinach (see Note)

1 medium (150 g/5.3 oz) avocado, sliced

Prepare the eggs the way you prefer (poached, soft-boiled, or fried; see page 10). Grease a large pan with the ghee and heat over medium heat. Place the sausage and bacon in the pan and cook for 5 to 10 minutes, until cooked through. (The sausage will take longer to cook.) Remove from the pan and keep warm.

Place the sliced mushrooms in the same pan you cooked the bacon and sausage in, and cook for 5 to 7 minutes, stirring frequently to prevent burning. Once cooked, take off the heat, and season with salt and pepper to taste. To serve, place the eggs, sausage, bacon, mushrooms, spinach, and avocado on a plate. Season with salt and pepper to taste.

To cook spinach, place it in a large pan and cook over medium heat for 1 to 2 minutes or until wilted, tossing gently with tongs. If all the spinach doesn't fit in the pan at once, add more in batches as it cooks down. Remove from the pan and set aside. Optionally, top each serving of cooked spinach with a tablespoon (15 g/0.5 oz) of butter.

NUTRITION FACTS PER SERVING

Total carbs: 13.3 g | Fiber: 8.2 g | Net carbs: 5.1 g | Protein: 25.2 g | Fat: 47.8 g | Energy: 565 kcal
Macronutrient ratio: Calories from carbs (4%), protein (18%), fat (78%)

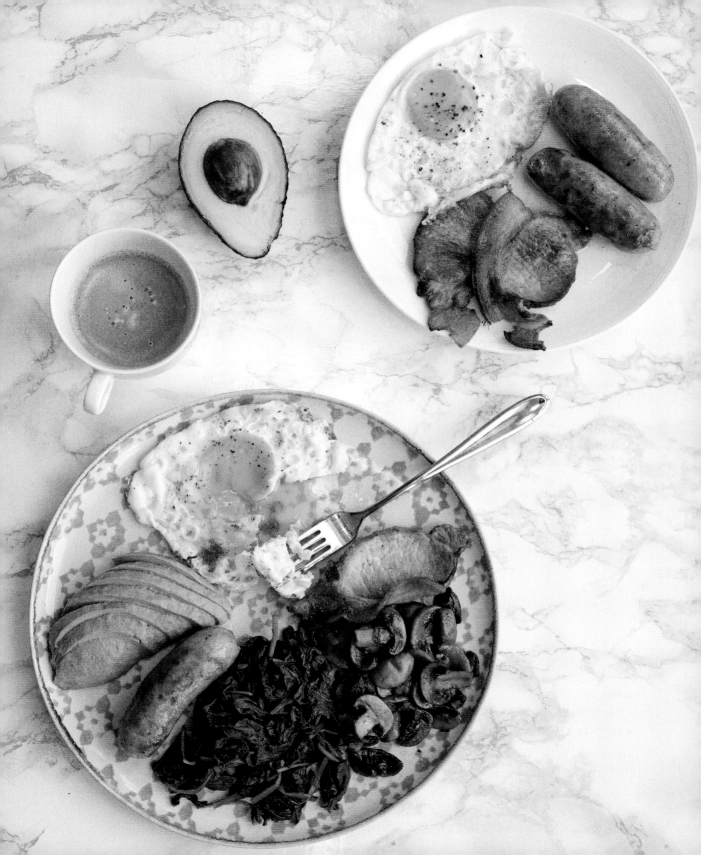

Quick Keto Cereal

When I crave something crispy for breakfast or a snack,
I make a few batches of this keto cereal. It's like grain-free granola:
tasty, convenient, and travel-friendly. And it lasts for weeks!

2 cups (120 g/4.2 oz) unsweetened flaked coconut

1 cup (90 g/3.2 oz) sliced almonds

⅓ cup (50 g/1.8 oz) chia seeds

½ cup (70 g/2.5 oz) hemp seeds

1 tablespoon (8 g/0.3 oz) ground cinnamon or vanilla powder

Pinch of salt

¼ cup (20 g/0.8 oz) unsweetened cacao powder

¼ cup (55 g/1.9 oz) virgin coconut oil, melted

Optional: 2 to 4 tablespoons (20 to 40 g/0.7 to 1.4 oz) erythritol or Swerve, or 5 to 15 drops liquid stevia extract

Preheat the oven to 300°F (150°C, or gas mark 2). Place all the ingredients in a mixing bowl and combine well. (If using stevia, mix it with the melted coconut oil before combining with the remaining ingredients.) Spread the mixture on a baking tray and transfer to the oven. Bake for 10 minutes, mixing the cereal halfway through. Remove from the oven and let the cereal cool down for a few minutes. Once it's completely cool, transfer to a jar or an airtight container. Store at room temperature for up to 1 month. Serve with coconut milk, almond milk, or full-fat yogurt.

⌐ If you can't eat nuts, try sunflower or pumpkin seeds instead of almonds.

NUTRITION FACTS PER SERVING (½ CUP/45 G/1.6 OZ CEREAL)

Total carbs: 11.4 g | Fiber: 8 g | Net carbs: 3.4 g | Protein: 8.7 g | Fat: 29.5 g | Energy: 321 kcal
Macronutrient ratio: Calories from carbs (4%), protein (11%), fat (85%)

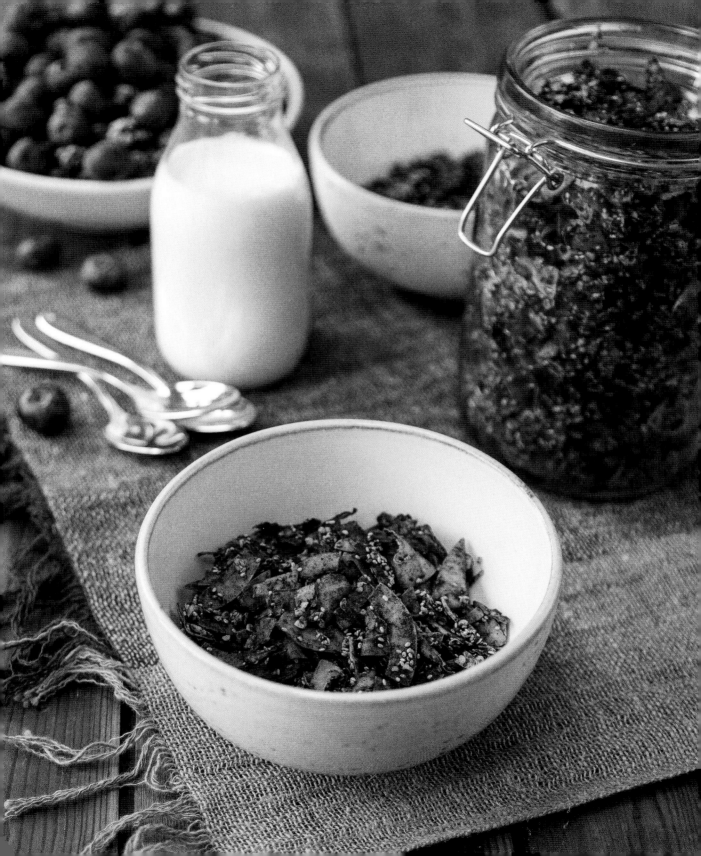

Pumpkin Pie "Noatmeal"

Chia seeds are a fantastic low-carb ingredient: you can use them in puddings, crackers, Raspberry Chia Jam (page 29), and even oatmeal. If you miss your morning oatmeal, you've got to try this recipe!

MAKES: 1 SERVING | HANDS-ON TIME: 5 MINUTES | OVERALL TIME: 10 TO 15 MINUTES

- 2 tablespoons (10 g/0.4 oz) unsweetened shredded coconut
- 2 tablespoons (8.5 g/0.3 oz) unsweetened flaked coconut or sliced almonds
- 2 tablespoons (16 g/0.6 oz) chia seeds
- 2 tablespoons (20 g/0.7 oz) hulled hemp seeds or sliced almonds
- ½ teaspoon pumpkin pie spice mix or cinnamon
- Optional: 1 tablespoon (10 g/0.4 oz) erythritol or Swerve, or 3 to 5 drops stevia extract
- 2 tablespoons (40 g/1.4 oz) unsweetened pumpkin purée
- ¼ cup (60 ml/2 oz) coconut milk or heavy whipping cream
- ¼ cup (60 ml/2 oz) hot or cold water
- Optional: 2 tablespoons (8.5 g/ 0.3 oz) toasted flaked coconut

Place all the dry ingredients in a serving bowl, plus the erythritol or stevia (if using). Add the pumpkin purée, coconut milk, and water. Stir, then let the mixture sit for 10 to 15 minutes before serving. Top with more coconut, if desired, and eat immediately, or make in batches and store in airtight containers in the fridge for up to 3 days.

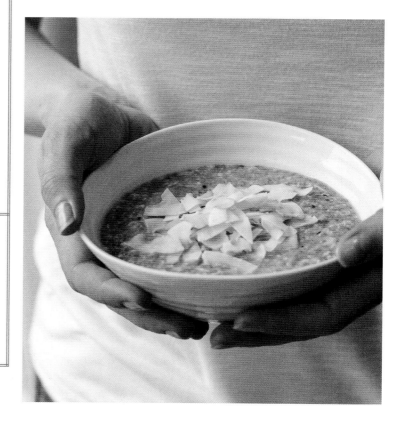

NUTRITION FACTS PER SERVING

Total carbs: 18.8 g | Fiber: 11.9 g
Net carbs: 6.9 g | Protein: 14.8 g
Fat: 34 g | Energy: 421 kcal
Macronutrient ratio: Calories from carbs (7%), protein (15%), fat (78%)

Chocolate Chip Pancakes

Nothing says "weekend" like these fluffy chocolate chip pancakes! They're the ultimate breakfast treat.

MAKES: 4 SERVINGS (8 MINI PANCAKES) | HANDS-ON TIME: 15 MINUTES | OVERALL TIME: 20 MINUTES

4 large pastured eggs

¼ cup (55 g/1.9 oz) virgin coconut oil or ghee, melted and divided

2 tablespoons (20 g/0.7 oz) erythritol

1 cup (100 g/3.5 oz) almond flour

½ teaspoon cinnamon or vanilla powder

1 teaspoon cream of tartar or apple cider vinegar

½ teaspoon baking soda

¼ cup (45 g/1.6 oz) dark chocolate chips (85% cacao or more), or roughly chopped dark chocolate

Crack the eggs into a bowl. Pour in the melted coconut oil, but reserve a small amount for greasing the pan. Whisk well. In another bowl, mix all the dry ingredients. Add the dry ingredients to the bowl with the eggs and mix well again. Stir in the dark chocolate chips.

Grease a large pan with the remaining coconut oil and heat over medium heat. Using a spoon or ladle, create small pancakes. (You can use pancake molds to create perfect shapes.) Lower the heat and cook for 3 to 5 minutes, or until the top of the pancake starts to firm up.

Flip the pancakes over and cook for an additional minute. Place the pancakes on a plate and keep warm in the oven until you've used up all the batter. Serve with butter, full-fat yogurt, or coconut cream.

Store leftover pancakes in an airtight container in the fridge for up to 5 days, or freeze for up to 3 months.

Make this recipe nut-free by substituting coconut flour for almond flour. Use ⅓ cup (40 g/1.4 oz) coconut flour instead of 1 cup (100 g/3.5 oz) almond flour.

NUTRITION FACTS PER SERVING (2 MINI PANCAKES)

Total carbs: 8.8 g | Fiber: 3.5 g | Net carbs: 5.3 g | Protein: 12.9 g | Fat: 40.4 g | Energy: 432 kcal
Macronutrient ratio: Calories from carbs (5%), protein (12%), fat (83%)

Cinnamon Roll Soufflé Pancake

Soufflé for breakfast? Sure! This fluffy, keto-friendly soufflé pancake is a light, airy, delicious riff on cinnamon rolls—minus the carbs. And, surprisingly, it takes just a few minutes to prepare.

MAKES: 1 SERVING | HANDS-ON TIME: 15 MINUTES | OVERALL TIME: 20 MINUTES

CINNAMON SWIRL FILLING:

1 tablespoon (15 g/0.5 oz) butter, ghee, or virgin coconut oil, melted

1 tablespoon (10 g/0.4 oz) powdered erythritol or Swerve

½ teaspoon cinnamon

PANCAKE:

3 large pastured eggs

¼ teaspoon cream of tartar or apple cider vinegar

1 tablespoon (10 g/0.4 oz) powdered erythritol or Swerve

2 tablespoons (16 g/0.6 oz) coconut flour

1 teaspoon ghee or virgin coconut oil

GLAZE:

1 tablespoon (15 ml/0.5 oz) heavy whipping cream or coconut milk

1 heaping tablespoon (28 g/1 oz) cream cheese, mascarpone, or coconut cream

⅛ teaspoon vanilla powder or cinnamon

1 teaspoon powdered erythritol or Swerve, or liquid stevia to taste

Preheat the oven to 400°F (200°C, or gas mark 6).

To make the cinnamon swirl filling, mix the melted butter with the erythritol and cinnamon. Set aside.

To make the pancake, separate the egg whites from the egg yolks. Mix the egg yolks with a fork. Using an electric mixer, beat the egg whites on medium-low speed. Continue for about 2 minutes until the whites become foamy. Add the cream of tartar and powdered erythritol. Keep beating until the egg whites form stiff peaks. Fold the egg yolks into the mixture using a silicone spatula. Sift in the coconut flour and gently combine with the egg mixture without deflating the egg whites.

Spread the pancake batter in a hot 8- to 9-inch (20 to 23 cm) skillet greased with the ghee. Use the rounded side of a teaspoon and draw a spiral-shaped swirl into the pancake, starting in the middle and ending at the edges. Then use the teaspoon to drizzle the prepared cinnamon filling into the swirl. Cook over low heat for about 5 minutes until the bottom of the pancake starts to brown. Remove from the burner and place under the broiler for about 5 minutes, or until the top is lightly browned.

Meanwhile, prepare the glaze. Heat the cream and cream cheese on high heat in the microwave for 10 to 15 seconds (or simply allow the mixture to come to room temperature beforehand). Mix with the vanilla powder and erythritol. Add a dash of water if it's too thick. Drizzle the glaze over the warm pancake and serve immediately.

NUTRITION FACTS PER SERVING

Total carbs: 9.3 g | Fiber: 3.6 g | Net carbs: 5.7 g | Protein: 24.1 g | Fat: 46.9 g | Energy: 553 kcal
Macronutrient ratio: Calories from carbs (4%), protein (18%), fat (78%)

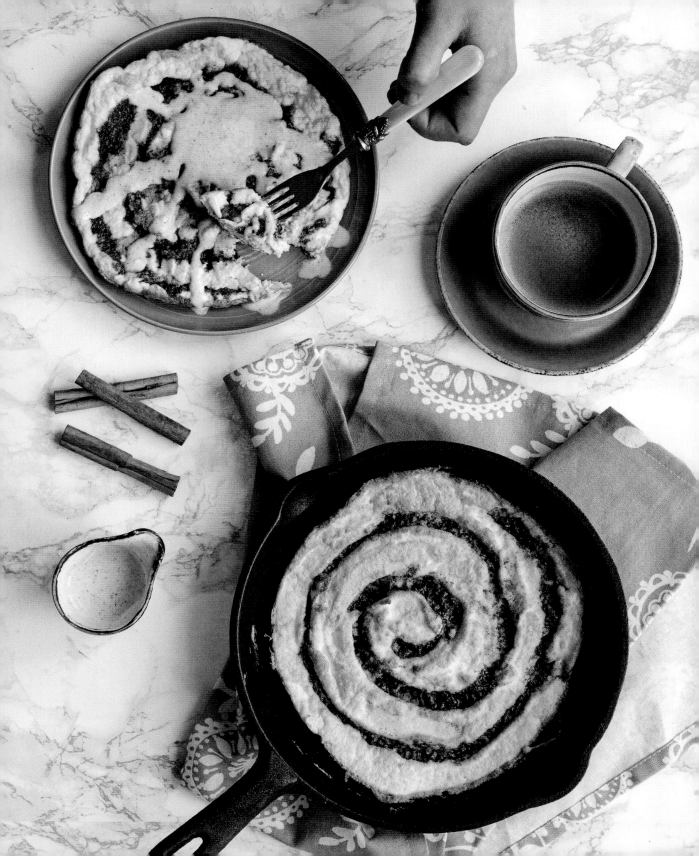

Chocolate-Berry Chia Parfaits

If you like to indulge your sweet tooth in the morning, you'll love this parfait: it's like having dessert for breakfast. You can make yours more (or less) sweet by adding a little low-carb sweetener, or just skip it altogether. Either way, the result is healthy, filling, and fun.

MAKES: 4 SERVINGS | HANDS-ON TIME: 10 MINUTES | OVERALL TIME: 30 MINUTES

CHIA LAYER:

¼ cup (32 g/1.1 oz) chia seeds

½ teaspoon cinnamon or vanilla powder

⅓ cup (80 ml/2.7 oz) coconut milk

½ cup (120 ml/4 oz) almond milk or water

Optional: 2 tablespoons (20 g/0.7 oz) powdered erythritol or Swerve, or 5 to 10 drops liquid stevia extract

CHOCOLATE LAYER:

1 cup (240 g/8.5 oz) creamed coconut milk (page 10) or mascarpone cheese

¼ cup (20 g/0.7 oz) unsweetened cocoa powder or raw cacao

2 tablespoons (20 g/0.7 oz) powdered erythritol or Swerve, or 5 to 10 drops liquid stevia extract

Pinch of salt

BERRY LAYER:

1¼ cups (150 g/5.3 oz) raspberries, fresh or frozen, or ½ cup (120 g/ 4.2 oz) Raspberry Chia Jam (page 29) plus 8 whole raspberries for serving

For the chia layer, place the chia seeds, cinnamon, coconut milk, and almond milk in a bowl. Optionally, add erythritol or stevia. Mix well and let the mixture sit for 15 to 20 minutes, or overnight.

For the chocolate layer, place the creamed coconut milk, cocoa powder, erythritol, and salt in a bowl. Mix with a whisk or an electric mixer until well combined.

If using fresh or frozen raspberries, place the raspberries in a bowl and mash with a fork. Reserve a few raspberries for topping. Or, measure out the Raspberry Chia Jam.

To assemble, place about 3 tablespoons (58 g/2 oz) of the chia seed layer in the bottom of each glass, add about ¼ cup (70 g/2.5 oz) of the chocolate layer, and top with about 2 tablespoons (38 g/1.3 oz) of the berry layer plus a few whole raspberries. Serve immediately, or seal with plastic wrap and refrigerate for up to 3 days.

NUTRITION FACTS PER SERVING

Total carbs: 15.8 g | Fiber: 8.5 g | Net carbs: 7.3 g | Protein: 5.8 g | Fat: 28.7 g | Energy: 312 kcal
Macronutrient ratio: Calories from carbs (9%), protein (8%), fat (83%)

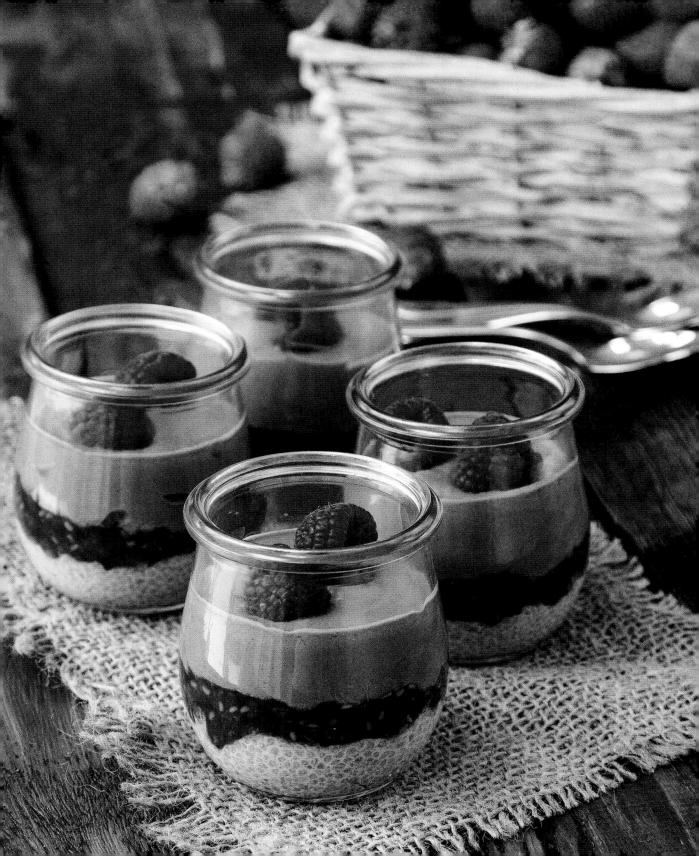

CHAPTER 4:

Snacks

When life gets busy, we're often tempted to reach for unhealthy options. Nowadays, high-carb foods—such as potato chips, crackers, and sugary bars often advertised as "health food"—are everywhere. It's not easy to avoid them, especially when you're caught hungry and unprepared. That's why it's so important to have quick, healthy snacks on hand. Apart from deviled eggs—a staple of low-carb diets—this chapter features quick, easy, tasty snack options, including keto-friendly crackers, savory dips, and crispy, spiced nuts. Dig in!

Omega-3 Deviled Eggs

Deviled eggs stuffed with fatty fish such as mackerel—which offers a healthy hit of omega-3 fatty acids—make a delicious keto-friendly snack or appetizer. Keep boiled eggs on hand in the fridge, and these deviled eggs will be ready in no time.

MAKES: 4 SERVINGS | HANDS-ON TIME: 10 MINUTES | OVERALL TIME: 15 MINUTES

4 large pastured eggs

½ cup (100 g/3.5 oz) canned mackerel, drained, or smoked skinless mackerel

2 tablespoons (30 g/1.1 oz) Mayonnaise (page 20)

2 tablespoons (30 ml/1 oz) fresh lemon juice

1 tablespoon (15 ml/0.5 oz) extra-virgin olive oil

Salt and pepper (omit if using smoked mackerel)

1 medium (15 g/0.5 oz) spring onion, sliced

First, hard-boil the eggs by following the instructions on page 8. Cut the eggs in half and carefully—without breaking the egg whites—spoon the egg yolks into a bowl. Set the whites aside.

Place the mackerel pieces, mayonnaise, lemon juice, and olive oil in a bowl. Mix with a fork. Season with salt and pepper, if necessary. Use a spoon or a small cookie scoop to fill in the egg white halves with the egg yolk mixture. Garnish with spring onion and serve, or store in an airtight container in the fridge for up to 2 days.

NUTRITION FACTS PER SERVING (2 DEVILED EGGS)

Total carbs: 1.1 g | Fiber: 0.1 g | Net carbs: 1 g | Protein: 11.8 g | Fat: 20.6 g | Energy: 237 kcal
Macronutrient ratio: Calories from carbs (2%), protein (20%), fat (78%)

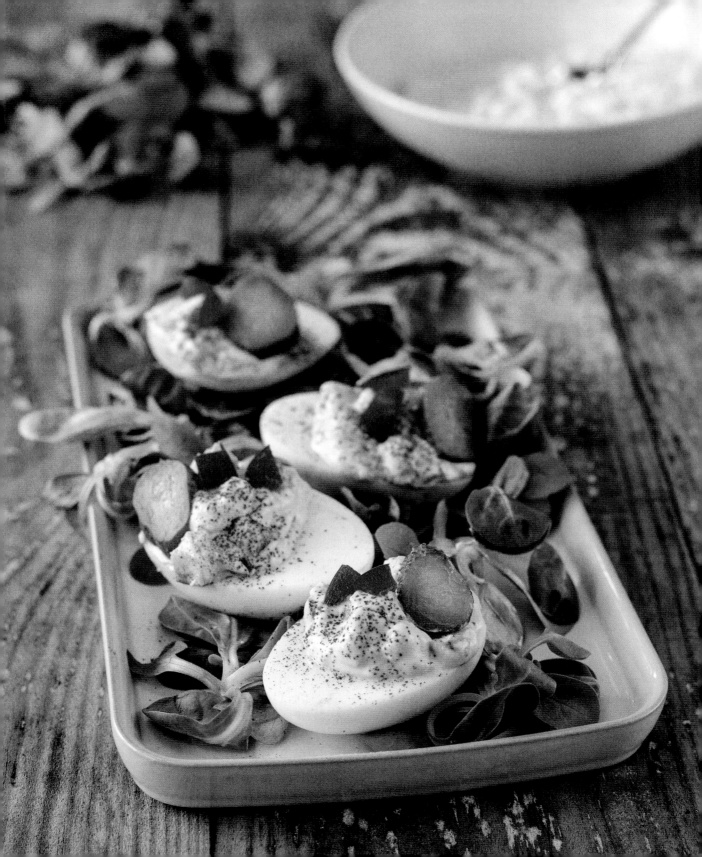

Southern Duck Deviled Eggs

These aren't your average deviled eggs. Made with duck eggs, which are bigger than chicken eggs (and more nutritious, too), they're extra-flavorful and very filling.

MAKES: 4 SERVINGS | HANDS-ON TIME: 10 MINUTES | OVERALL TIME: 20 MINUTES

4 duck eggs or jumbo chicken eggs

1 medium (40 g/1.4 oz) pickle

¼ cup (55 g/1.9 oz) Mayonnaise (page 20)

1 teaspoon Dijon mustard

1 tablespoon (15 ml/0.5 oz) pickle juice or fresh lemon juice

Salt and pepper

1 tablespoon (10 g/0.3 oz) diced red bell pepper

Pinch of paprika

First, hard-boil the eggs by following the instructions on page 8. Cut the eggs in half and carefully—without breaking the egg whites—spoon the egg yolks into a bowl. Set the whites aside.

Finely chop or slice the pickle, and reserve some for garnish. Add the mayonnaise, Dijon mustard, pickle juice, and pickles to the bowl with the egg yolks. Mix until well combined with a fork, and season with salt and pepper to taste.

Use a spoon or a small cookie scoop to fill in the egg white halves with the egg yolk mixture. Garnish with the reserved pickles, red pepper, and paprika. Serve, or place in an airtight container and refrigerate for up to 2 days.

NUTRITION FACTS PER SERVING (2 DEVILED EGGS)

Total carbs: 1.9 g | Fiber: 0.3 g | Net carbs: 1.6 g | Protein: 9.3 g | Fat: 21.1 g | Energy: 235 kcal
Macronutrient ratio: Calories from carbs (3%), protein (16%), fat (81%)

Crunchy Chile-Lime Nuts

I used to love the chile-lime nut mixes you can buy in grocery stores. But they're too high in carbs, and most of them have way too many additives. After some trial and error, though, I came up with a healthier version that tastes even better than the store-bought version!

MAKES: 12 SERVINGS (4 CUPS/480 G) | HANDS-ON TIME: 5 MINUTES | OVERALL TIME: 15 MINUTES

1 cup (100 g/3.5 oz) walnuts

1 cup (100 g/3.5 oz) pecans

1 cup (140 g/5 oz) almonds

1 cup (130 g/4.6 oz) macadamia nuts

1 teaspoon salt

½ teaspoon ground cumin

½ teaspoon paprika

¼ teaspoon cayenne pepper

¼ teaspoon black pepper

Optional: 1 tablespoon (10 g/0.3 oz) erythritol or Swerve, or 3 to 5 drops liquid stevia extract

1 tablespoon (15 ml/0.5 oz) lime juice

2 tablespoons (30 ml/1 oz) melted virgin coconut oil or ghee

Preheat the oven to 350°F (175°C, or gas mark 4). Place the nuts, preferably activated (page 10), in a mixing bowl. Add all the remaining ingredients. (If using stevia, mix it with the lime juice before adding it to the nuts.) Mix until well combined and all the nuts are coated with the spices. Spread the nuts in a single layer on a baking sheet lined with parchment paper. Roast for 8 to 12 minutes, mixing the nuts with a spatula halfway through. Remove from the oven and let cool. Store in an airtight container for up to 1 month.

If possible, use soaked and dehydrated nuts for this recipe. You can use any of your favorite nuts here; just avoid pistachios and cashews because they are relatively high in carbs. You can even make this a nut-free snack by using unsweetened flaked coconut and mixed seeds—such as sunflower, pumpkin, sesame, and hemp seeds—in place of the nuts.

NUTRITION FACTS PER SERVING (ABOUT ⅓ CUP/40 G/1.4 OZ)

Total carbs: 6.5 g | Fiber: 3.8 g | Net carbs: 2.8 g | Protein: 5.4 g | Fat: 27.7 g | Energy: 277 kcal
Macronutrient ratio: Calories from carbs (4%), protein (8%), fat (88%)

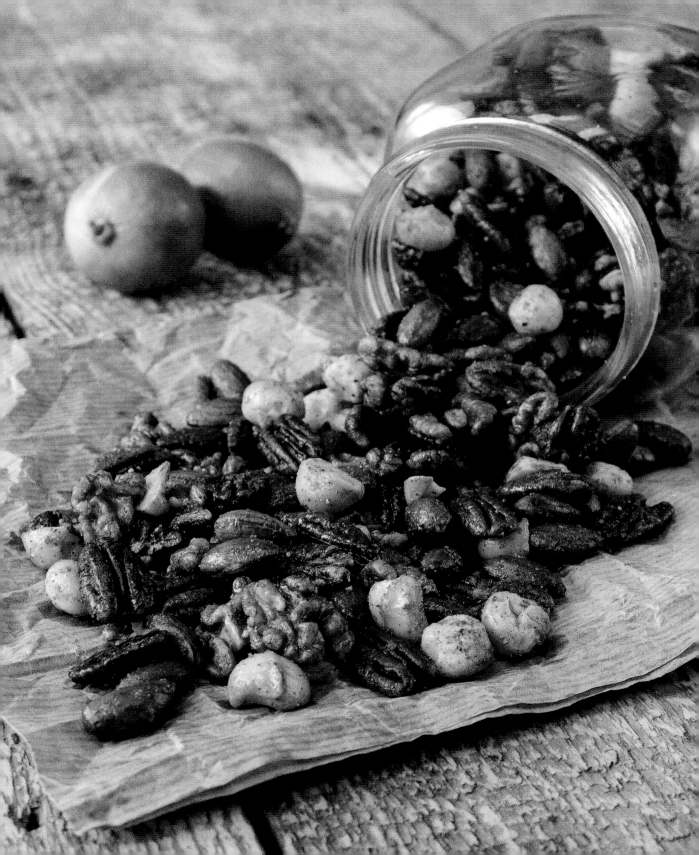

Speedy Keto Crackers

Crackers don't have to be high in carbs. These thin, crispy crackers are perfect for healthy snacking: dip them in guacamole or Creamy Crab Dip (page 64), or top them with butter or Easy Chicken Liver Pâté (page 65).

MAKES: 12 SERVINGS (24 CRACKERS) | HANDS-ON TIME: 10 MINUTES | OVERALL TIME: 30 MINUTES

½ cup (75 g/2.6 oz) flax meal

¼ cup (38 g/1.3 oz) chia seeds

¼ cup (36 g/1.3 oz) sesame seeds

¼ cup (32 g/1.1 oz) pumpkin seeds

½ cup (45 g/1.6 oz) grated Parmesan cheese

½ teaspoon salt

½ teaspoon coarse black pepper

½ teaspoon red pepper flakes

½ cup (120 ml/4 oz) water

Preheat the oven to 400°F (200°C, or gas mark 6). Place all the ingredients into a bowl and mix until well combined. Place the dough on top of a nonstick baking mat or a piece of strong parchment paper.

Place a piece of plastic wrap or parchment paper on top of the dough. Use a rolling pin to roll out the dough into a 12 x 16-inch (30 x 40 cm) rectangle. The dough should be no more than ⅛ inch (25 mm) thick. Using a pizza cutter or a large knife, pre-cut the dough into 24 equal squares. (Pre-cutting the dough will make the crackers easy to slice once they crisp up.)

Transfer the baking mat to a baking sheet and bake for 18 to 20 minutes. Remove from the oven. Cut or break the dough into the pre-cut crackers. Let the crackers cool so that they become crisp. Store in an airtight container at room temperature for up to 2 weeks.

NUTRITION FACTS PER SERVING (2 CRACKERS)

Total carbs: 4.4 g | Fiber: 3.4 g | Net carbs: 1 g | Protein: 4.5 g | Fat: 7.5 g | Energy: 97 kcal
Macronutrient ratio: Calories from carbs (4%), protein (20%), fat (76%)

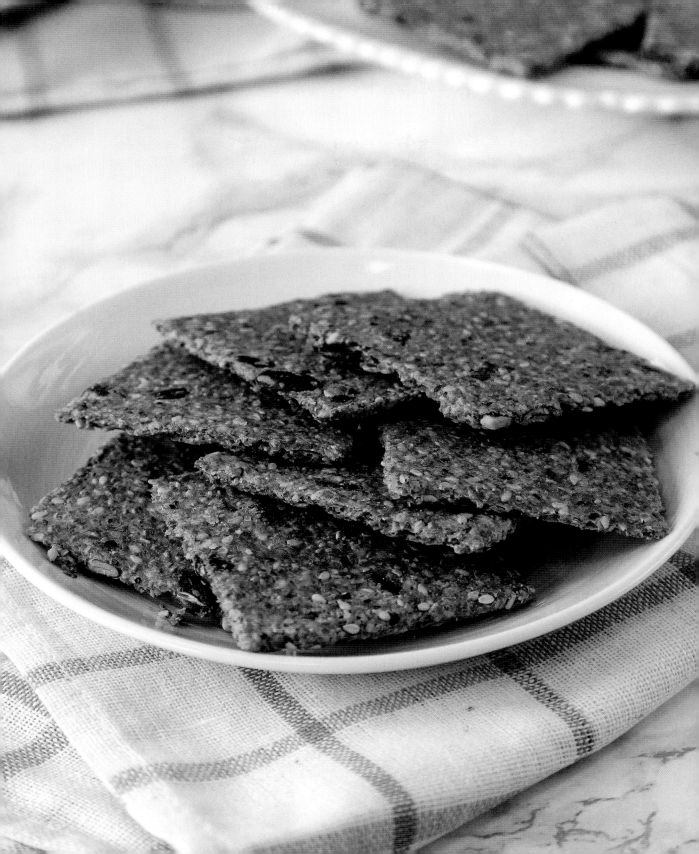

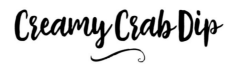

Creamy Crab Dip

This creamy appetizer takes just minutes to make. It's perfect for parties—
or just everyday snacking—alongside a handful of low-carb crackers or veggies.

MAKES: 8 SERVINGS (4 CUPS/800 G/28.2 OZ) | HANDS-ON TIME: 5 MINUTES | OVERALL TIME: 5 MINUTES

1 pound (450 g) crabmeat, cooked or canned

1 cup (240 g/8.5 oz) full-fat cream cheese

⅓ cup (75 g/2.6 oz) Mayonnaise (page 20)

1 tablespoon (15 g/0.5 oz) Sriracha sauce

1 teaspoon Dijon mustard

1 clove garlic, minced

2 tablespoons (30 ml/1 oz) fresh lemon or lime juice

2 teaspoons (5 g/0.2 oz) Old Bay seasoning

3 medium (45 g/1.6 oz) spring onions, sliced

3 tablespoons (12 g/0.4 oz) chopped fresh parsley

Salt and pepper

Combine all the ingredients in a mixing bowl. Season with salt and pepper to taste. Serve immediately, or store in an airtight container in the fridge for up to 3 days. Try this dip with my Speedy Keto Crackers (page 62).

 This recipe works well with canned or fresh crabmeat. You can even replace some of the crabmeat with cooked, chopped shrimp or cooked, flaked white fish, such as pollock, haddock, or cod.

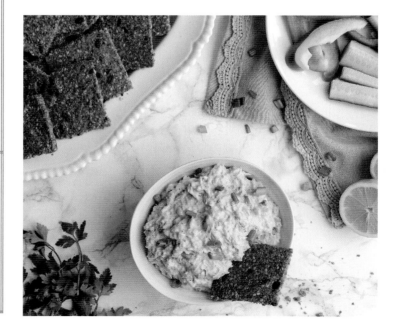

NUTRITION FACTS PER SERVING (½ CUP/100 G/3.5 OZ)

Total carbs: 2.5 g | Fiber: 0.4 g
Net carbs: 2.1 g | Protein: 15.2 g
Fat: 18.8 g | Energy: 224 kcal
Macronutrient ratio: Calories from carbs (4%), protein (25%), fat (71%)

Easy Chicken Liver Pâté

Organ meats should be a part of every healthy diet. They're rich in vitamins and minerals, especially vitamin A, vitamin B_{12}, folic acid, and iron. (Contrary to popular belief, liver does not store toxins: it's perfectly safe to eat.) If you're new to offal, this quick-and-easy pâté is a great place to start.

MAKES: 9 SERVINGS (3 CUPS/720 G/25.4 OZ) | HANDS-ON TIME: 15 MINUTES | OVERALL TIME: 20 MINUTES

2 tablespoons (30 g/1.1 oz) ghee or duck fat, divided

1.1 pounds (500 g) chicken or turkey livers, chopped

1 medium (110 g/3.9 oz) white or yellow onion, diced

2 cloves garlic, minced

⅓ cup (76 g/2.7 oz) butter or ghee

1 tablespoon (2 g/0.07 oz) fresh thyme (or 1 teaspoon dried)

1 tablespoon (5 g/0.2 oz) fresh oregano (or 1 teaspoon dried)

1 teaspoon Dijon mustard

Salt and pepper

Heat 1 tablespoon (15 g/0.5 oz) of the ghee in a pan and add the chopped livers. Cook for about 3 minutes, until they're browned on the outside but still pink inside. Transfer the livers to a blender and set aside.

Place the remaining 1 tablespoon (15 g/0.5 oz) ghee into a clean pan. Add the onion and garlic. Cook over medium heat for about 10 minutes, stirring frequently. Add the cooked onion-garlic mixture to the blender with the chicken livers. Add the butter, thyme, oregano, and Dijon mustard. Season with salt and epper to taste, and pulse until smooth.

Eat immediately with freshly cut vegetables or Speedy Keto Crackers (page 62). To store, transfer to an airtight container and refrigerate for up to 2 days. To keep the pâté for up to 3 months, divide it into small containers and pour a layer of fat—such as lard, ghee, or tallow—on top of each to seal it.

NUTRITION FACTS PER SERVING (⅓ CUP/80 G/2.8 OZ)

Total carbs: 1.9 g | Fiber: 0.4 g | Net carbs: 1.5 g | Protein: 9.7 g | Fat: 12.9 g | Energy: 163 kcal
Macronutrient ratio: Calories from carbs (4%), protein (24%), fat (72%)

CHAPTER 5:

Quick Lunches

Finding healthy, filling lunch options when you're out and about is nearly impossible, isn't it? Your options are limited to little more than sandwiches, cold pasta meals, and burgers from local fast food chains—or those sad, ineffectual, miniature salads that are served with low-fat dressings and painfully small amounts of meat, fish, or cheese. Luckily, it's easy to prepare quick, lunchbox-friendly meals at home. And this chapter will show you how. From healthy wraps and rolls to frittatas and egg muffins, the no-fuss recipes here suit even the busiest lifestyles. You're good to go!

Eggplant Parma Ham Rolls

Eggplant, also known as aubergine, is a great source of phytochemicals and antioxidants, most of which are found in its lovely dark purple skin. When sliced thinly and baked, eggplants are great for using as wraps. And, with their Mediterranean pedigree, they're a delicious match for goat cheese, pesto, and Parma ham.

MAKES: 3 SERVINGS (6 ROLLS) | HANDS-ON TIME: 15 MINUTES | OVERALL TIME: 30 MINUTES

EGGPLANT SLICES:

1 medium (250 g/8.8 oz) eggplant

2 tablespoons (30 g/1.1 oz) ghee, melted, or extra-virgin olive oil

¼ teaspoon salt, or to taste

Pepper

FILLING:

5.3 oz (150 g) soft goat cheese

2 tablespoons (30 g/1.1 oz) Avocado and Kale Pesto (page 19)

LEMON VINAIGRETTE:

2 tablespoons (30 ml/1 oz) extra-virgin olive oil

1 tablespoon (15 ml/0.5 oz) fresh lemon juice

1 teaspoon balsamic vinegar

SERVE WITH:

6 slices (85 g/3 oz) Parma ham

6 cups (180 g/6.3 oz) fresh spinach or other leafy greens

Fresh basil and black pepper

To make the eggplant, preheat the oven to 400°F (200°C, or gas mark 6). Cut the eggplant lengthwise into 6 slices of about ½ inch (1 cm) each. Place on a baking sheet lined with parchment paper. Brush the eggplant on both sides with melted ghee. Season with salt and pepper. Transfer to the oven and bake for 15 to 18 minutes, until cooked through. Set aside to cool.

Meanwhile, to make the filling, place the goat cheese and pesto in a bowl. Mix until well combined.

To make the vinaigrette, in another bowl, combine the olive oil, lemon juice, and balsamic vinegar.

To assemble the rolls, place a slice of Parma ham onto each slice of the eggplant, spread with about 2 tablespoons of the goat cheese filling, and roll them up. Serve on a bed of spinach (2 cups [60 g/2.1 oz] per serving). Drizzle with the lemon vinaigrette, and garnish with basil leaves and black pepper. Serve immediately, or store the eggplant rolls (without spinach) in an airtight container in the fridge for up to 3 days.

NUTRITION FACTS PER SERVING (2 ROLLS + GREENS)

Total carbs: 8.6 g | Fiber: 4.1 g | Net carbs: 4.5 g | Protein: 19.5 g | Fat: 39.8 g | Energy: 462 kcal
Macronutrient ratio: Calories from carbs (4%), protein (17%), fat (79%)

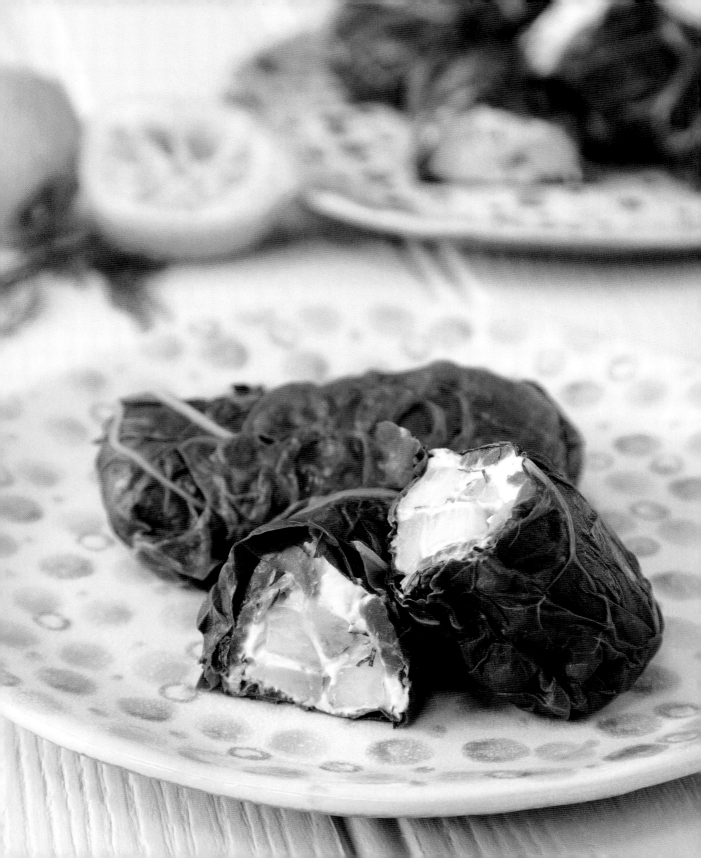

Smoked Salmon Chard Wraps

An easy-to-prepare lunchbox meal, these wraps have the perfect balance of carbs, protein, and healthy fats.

MAKES: 2 SERVINGS (4 WRAPS) | HANDS-ON TIME: 10 MINUTES | OVERALL TIME: 10 MINUTES

4 to 8 chard or collard leaves (120 g/4.2 oz)

½ medium (100 g/3.5 oz) cucumber

1 small (100 g/3.5 oz) avocado

3.5 ounces (100 g) smoked salmon

1 tablespoon (15 ml/0.5 oz) fresh lemon juice

½ cup (120 g/4.2 oz) full-fat cream cheese

1 tablespoon (4 g/0.1 oz) freshly chopped dill or chives

Bring a large pot of water to a boil, and blanch the chard leaves for 20 to 30 seconds. Using tongs, immediately remove the leaves from the boiling water and plunge them into a bowl of ice water. Drain and dry the leaves on a clean dish towel or paper towels. Place them, one at a time, on a chopping board, cut the stems off, and set aside. (Reserve the stems for the Sausage and Turnip Hash [page 38] or the Mexican Hash [page 40].)

Peel and cut the cucumber into thin strips. Peel and slice the avocado, and set aside. Drizzle the salmon with lemon juice.

To assemble, place the salmon in the center of 1 or 2 chard leaves. Spoon the cream cheese on top of the salmon. Add the dill, cucumber, and avocado. Make sure you leave some space on each side. Fold the long sides of the leaf over the filling. Roll up the chard wrap tightly. Secure with a toothpick, if necessary. Eat immediately or store in the fridge for up to 2 days.

NUTRITION FACTS PER SERVING (2 WRAPS)

Total carbs: 10.2 g | Fiber: 4.8 g | Net carbs: 5.3 g | Protein: 15.8 g | Fat: 26.5 g | Energy: 305 kcal
Macronutrient ratio: Calories from carbs (6%), protein (20%), fat (74%)

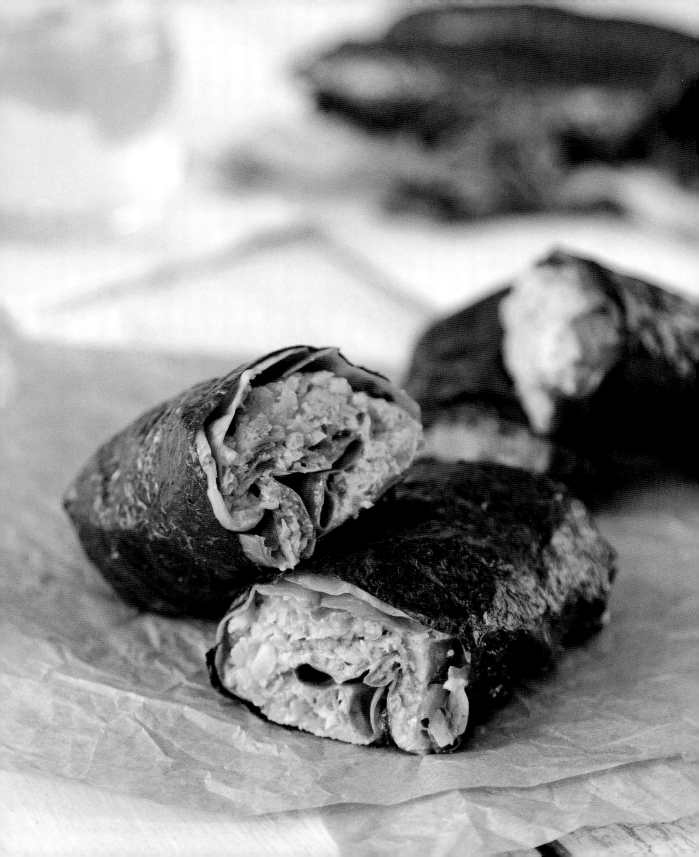

Sardine and Turmeric Nori Wraps

Sardines are high in healthy omega-3 fatty acids and low in mercury. And, as a bonus, they're one of the most sustainable fish on the market. So go ahead and enjoy them! Canned sardines are as good as fresh ones—just make sure you get yours in a BPA-free can.

MAKES: 4 SERVINGS (8 WRAPS) | HANDS-ON TIME: 15 MINUTES | OVERALL TIME: 20 MINUTES

2 tablespoons (30 g/1.1 oz) ghee or virgin coconut oil

1 small (70 g/2.5 oz) white onion, finely chopped

1 clove garlic, minced

2 cups (240 g/8.5 oz) uncooked cauliflower rice (page 8)

1 teaspoon ground turmeric

Salt and pepper

6.3 ounces (180 g) canned sardines, drained

¼ cup (55 g/1.9 oz) Mayonnaise (page 20)

1 tablespoon (15 g/0.5 oz) Sriracha sauce

1 tablespoon (15 ml/0.5 oz) fresh lemon juice

4 nori sheets

8 chard leaves (120 g/4.2 oz)

Grease a medium pan with the ghee. Add the onion and garlic. Cook over medium heat until fragrant, 3 to 5 minutes. Add the cauliflower rice, turmeric, and salt and pepper to taste. Cook for 5 to 7 minutes, then transfer to a bowl to cool.

In a separate bowl, using a fork, shred the sardines. Mix with the mayonnaise, Sriracha, and lemon juice. Season with salt and pepper to taste. Cut each nori sheet in half. Cut the stems off the chard leaves. (Reserve the stems for the Sausage and Turnip Hash [page 38] or the Mexican Hash [page 40].)

To assemble, place the nori sheets, one at a time, on a chopping board. Add 1 chard leaf, about 2 tablespoons of the cauliflower rice filling, and about 2 tablespoons of the sardine filling. Make sure you leave some space on each side of the nori sheet. Fold the long sides of the nori over the filling. Roll the wrap tight and wet the edges of the nori to help it hold together. Secure with a toothpick, if necessary. Store in the fridge for up to 2 days.

NUTRITION FACTS PER SERVING (2 WRAPS)

Total carbs: 7.8 g | Fiber: 3 g | Net carbs: 4.7 g | Protein: 14.2 g | Fat: 24.7 g | Energy: 302 kcal
Macronutrient ratio: Calories from carbs (7%), protein (19%), fat (74%)

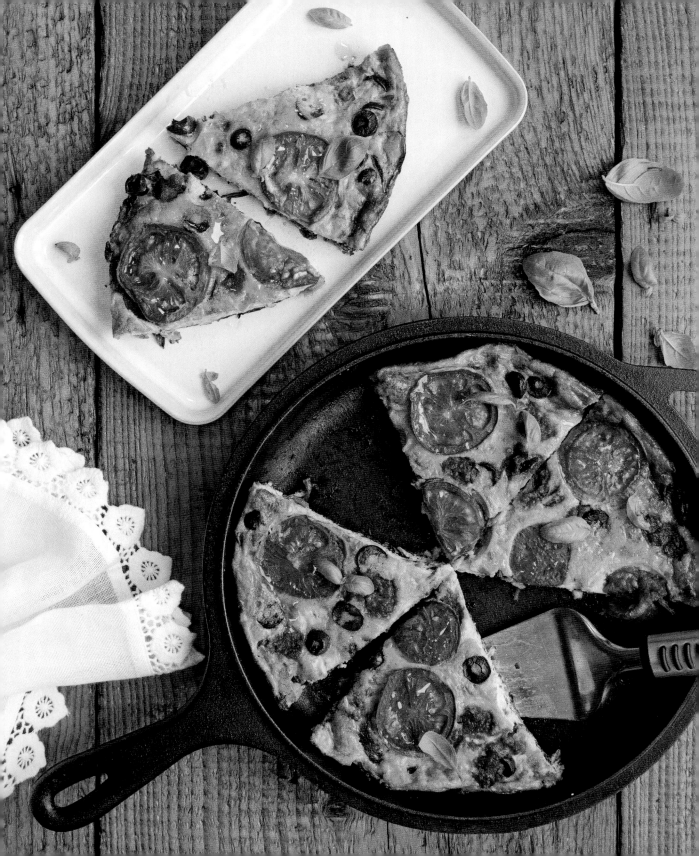

Pizza Frittata

This simple frittata takes its inspiration from Margherita- and Florentine-style pizzas—except, of course, it's low-carb and grain-free. Laden with cheese and vegetables, it's sure to keep you going until dinnertime.

MAKES: 3 SERVINGS (6 SLICES) | HANDS-ON TIME: 20 MINUTES | OVERALL TIME: 30 MINUTES

1 tablespoon (15 g/0.5 oz) ghee or lard

1 small (70 g/2.5 oz) white or yellow onion, chopped

4 ounces (112 g) fresh or cooked spinach

6 large pastured eggs

⅓ cup (80 g/2.8 oz) sugar-free marinara sauce, divided (see Tip)

⅓ cup (30 g/1.1 oz) grated Parmesan cheese, divided

1 cup (112 g/4 oz) grated mozzarella cheese, divided

2 medium (150 g/5.3 oz) tomatoes, sliced

¼ cup (25 g/0.9 oz) sliced olives

1 tablespoon (15 ml/0.5 oz) extra-virgin olive oil

Fresh basil

Grease a pan with the ghee and add the onion. Cook over medium-high heat for 2 to 3 minutes, or until fragrant. Add the spinach and cook for no more than 1 minute. (If you're using fresh spinach, you may need to add it in batches until it cooks down.)

Preheat the broiler. Crack the eggs into a bowl and beat with a fork. Add the marinara, grated Parmesan, and mozzarella. (Reserve some marinara sauce and cheese for topping.) Pour the egg mixture into the pan and lower the heat to medium-low. Cook until the top starts to firm up and the edges are turning opaque, about 8 to 10 minutes. Top with the reserved marinara and cheese, tomatoes, and olives. Place under the broiler for 5 to 7 minutes to crisp up the top. Let the frittata cool slightly and cut it into 6 pieces. Top with extra-virgin olive oil and fresh basil just before serving.

⌒ Make your own marinara sauce. For 2 cups of marinara sauce, place 1 cup (150 g/5.3 oz) chopped tomatoes, ½ cup (20 g/0.7 oz) fresh basil, 2 cloves garlic, 1 small (30 g/1.1 oz) shallot or white onion, ¼ cup (60 g/2.1 oz) tomato paste, ¼ cup (60 ml/2 oz) extra-virgin olive oil, ¼ teaspoon salt and pepper to taste into a blender. Pulse until smooth.

NUTRITION FACTS PER SERVING (⅓ FRITTATA, 2 SLICES)

Total carbs: 9.6 g | Fiber: 2.5 g | Net carbs: 7.1 g | Protein: 28.1 g | Fat: 35.9 g | Energy: 473 kcal
Macronutrient ratio: Calories from carbs (6%), protein (24%), fat (70%)

Taco Frittata

This frittata features the best parts of a taco—onion, garlic, punchy seasoning, cheese, and olives—all in one low-carb package. Instead of using beans here, which aren't low-carb or paleo-friendly, one of my blog readers suggested I use eggplant instead. To my surprise, it worked wonderfully!

MAKES: 3 SERVINGS (6 SLICES) | HANDS-ON TIME: 20 MINUTES | OVERALL TIME: 30 MINUTES

2 tablespoons (30 g/1.1 oz) ghee or lard

1 small (70 g/2.5 oz) white onion, chopped

½ medium (125 g/4.4 oz) eggplant

8.8 ounces (250 g) ground beef

1 tablespoon (8 g/0.3 oz) taco seasoning

2 tablespoons (30 ml/1 oz) water

6 large pastured eggs

½ cup (60 g/2.1 oz) grated Cheddar cheese

¼ cup (25 g/0.9 oz) sliced black olives

Heat a large pan greased with ghee over medium heat. Add the onion and cook until fragrant, about 3 minutes. Meanwhile, dice the eggplant into ½-inch (1 cm) pieces. Add to the pan and cook for another 5 minutes. Add the ground beef, taco seasoning, and water, and cook for 3 to 5 minutes, until the meat is browned on all sides and the eggplant is tender.

Preheat the broiler. Crack the eggs into a bowl and whisk with a fork. Add the Cheddar cheese and sliced olives to the pan, then pour in the whisked eggs. Stir to combine and cook until firm, about 10 minutes. Finally, place the pan under the broiler and cook for 5 minutes to crisp up the top.

Let the frittata cool slightly and cut it into 6 pieces. Once completely cooled, store in the fridge in an airtight container for up to 5 days. Serve with sour cream, diced avocado, and Fresh Tomato Salsa (page 31).

NUTRITION FACTS PER SERVING (⅓ FRITTATA, 2 SLICES)

Total carbs: 6.9 g | Fiber: 2.5 g | Net carbs: 4.4 g | Protein: 32.7 g | Fat: 45 g | Energy: 569 kcal
Macronutrient ratio: Calories from carbs (3%), protein (24%), fat (73%)

Green Omelet Wraps

These wraps are great lunchbox fillers, and they're incredibly versatile. Short on protein? Add some smoked salmon or chicken. Need a dose of healthy fats? Stuff your wrap with a few slices of avocado. The possibilities are endless.

MAKES: 1 SERVING | HANDS-ON TIME: 10 MINUTES | OVERALL TIME: 15 MINUTES

3 large pastured eggs

1 tablespoon (15 g/0.5 oz) Avocado and Kale Pesto (page 19)

1 cup (30 g/1.1 oz) fresh spinach, or 1 ounce (28 g) cooked spinach

1 tablespoon (15 g/0.5 oz) ghee or lard

⅓ cup (50 g/1.8 oz) crumbled feta (or crisped-up bacon, if you're dairy-free)

4 olives, sliced, or 1 sliced sun-dried tomato

Salt and pepper

Crack the eggs into a bowl, add the pesto, and whisk with a fork. Roughly chop the spinach (if using cooked spinach, drain it well first). Add the spinach to the bowl with the eggs. Pour the egg mixture into a hot pan greased with the ghee. Add the feta and olives, and cook for a few minutes over medium heat until the top starts to firm up.

Slide the omelet onto a chopping board lined with parchment paper. Holding the omelet and the parchment paper together, roll the omelet up tightly. (The parchment paper will prevent you from burning your fingers.) Remove the paper from the wrap. Serve immediately as is, or stuff the wrap with chicken, avocado, or other fillings of your choice. Or, store in an airtight container (without fillings) in the fridge for up to 3 days.

NUTRITION FACTS PER SERVING

Total carbs: 5.9 g | Fiber: 1.3 g
Net carbs: 4.6 g | Protein: 27.5 g
Fat: 51.6 g | Energy: 600 kcal
Macronutrient ratio: Calories from carbs (3%), protein (19%), fat (78%)

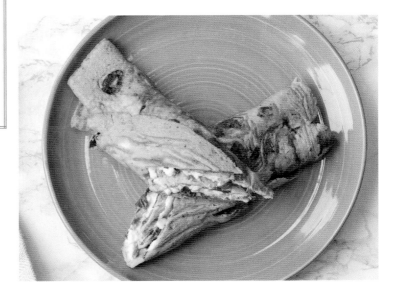

Chorizo Egg Muffins

Egg muffins are a snap to make. They're also easy to take in lunchboxes or to grab as you're running out the door. What could be more convenient? Have a batch at the ready in the fridge.

MAKES: 5 SERVINGS (10 MUFFINS) | HANDS-ON TIME: 10 MINUTES | OVERALL TIME: 30 MINUTES

3.5 ounces (100 g) Spanish chorizo or pepperoni

3.5 ounces (100 g) chopped par-boiled kale (page 11) or fresh kale

6 large pastured eggs

1 cup (200 g/7.1 oz) unsweetened pumpkin purée

Salt and pepper

Optional: ½ cup (60 g/2.1 oz) grated Manchego or Cheddar cheese

Optional: Sriracha sauce, greens, sliced avocado

Preheat the oven to 360°F (180°C, or gas mark 4). Dice the chorizo and place on a hot dry pan. Cook for 1 to 2 minutes to release the juices and crisp it up. Add the parboiled kale and cook for another minute. (If using fresh kale: Cover with a lid and cook for 5 to 7 minutes over medium-low heat.) Remove from the heat and set aside.

Crack the eggs into a bowl and mix with the pumpkin purée. Add the chorizo and kale. Season with salt and pepper, and mix until combined. Add the grated cheese (if using).

Spoon the mixture into a muffin tray (a silicone tray works best). Use a ladle to distribute the mixture evenly among 10 muffin cups. (Or, bake in a skillet to make a frittata.) Bake for 20 to 25 minutes, and set aside to cool slightly before serving. Serve with Sriracha sauce, greens, or sliced avocado, if you like. Store in the fridge in an airtight container for up to 5 days.

NUTRITION FACTS PER SERVING (2 MUFFINS)

Total carbs: 5.3 g | Fiber: 1.7 g | Net carbs: 3.6 g | Protein: 13.2 g | Fat: 13.7 g | Energy: 198 kcal
Macronutrient ratio: Calories from carbs (8%), protein (28%), fat (65%)

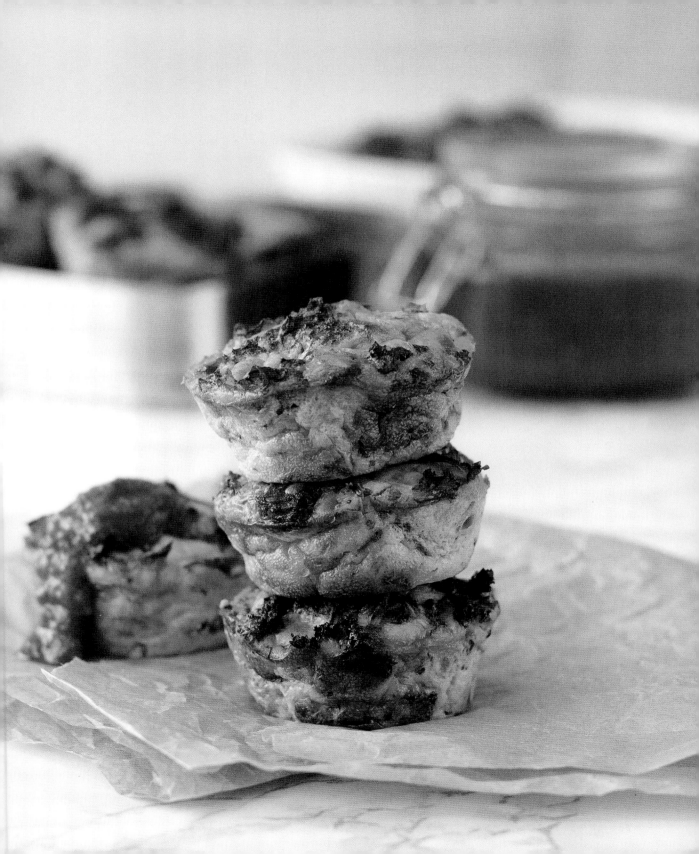

Quick Egg Muffin in a Mug, Two Ways

Incredibly speedy and convenient—all you need is a mug and a microwave—egg muffins are blank canvases, so feel free to get creative with them. These are just two of the many ways you can prepare this quick keto meal.

MAKES: 1 SERVING | HANDS-ON TIME: 5 MINUTES | OVERALL TIME: 5 MINUTES

2 large pastured eggs

2 ounces (56 g) cooked spinach, or parboiled chard or kale (page 11)

1 tablespoon (15 g/0.5 oz) softened ghee or butter

Salt and pepper

VEGETARIAN EGG MUFFIN:

2 ounces (56 g) goat cheese or other soft cheese

1 tablespoon (3 g/0.1 oz) fresh chives or spring onion

HAM & CHEESE EGG MUFFIN:

1 ounce (28 g) ham or bacon, sliced

1 ounce (28 g) grated or diced Cheddar cheese

Place all the ingredients into a mug. The mug should be no more than two-thirds full or it will overflow. Cook it in the microwave for 2½ to 3 minutes, checking halfway through to make sure the mug isn't overflowing. Serve immediately.

You can easily make this quick meal at work. Just store all the ingredients in an airtight container. Place everything in a mug, crack in the egg, and cook in the microwave. Lunch is served!

Contrary to popular belief, most studies show that microwaves don't decrease the nutritional value of foods. In fact, some research demonstrates that cooking or reheating your food in a microwave can preserve more nutrients than other cooking methods. And they don't emit harmful radiation, either: that's another myth. Microwaves produce nonionizing radiation, which is the same type of radiation produced by toasters, TVs, and cell phones.

NUTRITION FACTS PER SERVING (VEGETARIAN MUFFIN)

Total carbs: 3.4 g | Fiber: 1.7 g | Net carbs: 1.6 g | Protein: 27 g | Fat: 41.8 g | Energy: 503 kcal
Macronutrient ratio: Calories from carbs (1%), protein (22%), fat (77%)

NUTRITION FACTS PER SERVING (HAM & CHEESE MUFFIN)

Total carbs: 3.7 g | Fiber: 1.7 g | Net carbs: 2 g | Protein: 26.4 g | Fat: 35.3 g | Energy: 440 kcal
Macronutrient ratio: Calories from carbs (2%), protein (24%), fat (74%)

Portobello Tuna Melts

Who says you need bread to make tuna melts? Not me!
There's a healthier alternative that tastes even better: portobello mushrooms.
These open-faced "sandwiches" are hearty and flavorful.

MAKES: 2 SERVINGS | HANDS-ON TIME: 15 MINUTES | OVERALL TIME: 20 MINUTES

MUSHROOM BUNS:

4 portobello (300 g/10.6 oz) or large flat mushrooms

Salt and pepper

1 tablespoon (15 g/0.5 oz) ghee or lard

FILLING:

2 cans (225 g/8 oz) tuna, drained

¼ cup (55 g/1.9 oz) Mayonnaise (page 20)

2 tablespoons (30 ml/1 oz) fresh lemon juice

1 medium (40 g/1.4 oz) celery stalk, finely chopped

2 medium (30 g/1.1 oz) spring onions, sliced

2 tablespoons (8 g/0.3 oz) chopped parsley or chives, divided

TOPPING:

1 large (150 g/5.3 oz) tomato

4 slices (80 g/2.8 oz) Swiss, provolone, or Cheddar cheese

2 tablespoons (30 ml/1 oz) extra-virgin olive oil

To make the mushroom buns, clean the mushrooms with a damp paper towel. Remove the stems and reserve for another recipe (such as Good-for-Your-Gut-Scrambles, page 44). Season the mushrooms with salt and pepper. Place in a hot ovenproof pan greased with ghee, bottom-side up. Cook for 1 to 2 minutes, then flip over. Cover with a lid and cook for 5 to 7 minutes, or until tender. When done, turn the mushrooms bottom-side up and remove from the heat.

To make the tuna filling, place the drained tuna into a bowl and add the mayonnaise, lemon juice, celery, spring onions, and parsley. (Reserve some parsley for garnish.) Mix, and season with salt and pepper to taste. Preheat the broiler.

To make the topping, cut the tomato into 4 slices. To assemble, divide the mixture into 4 parts and spoon it on top of each cooked mushroom. Place a slice of tomato and a slice of cheese on top of each. Place under the broiler for 3 to 5 minutes, or until the cheese melts. Sprinkle with the reserved chopped parsley, and drizzle with the olive oil. Serve immediately.

NUTRITION FACTS PER SERVING (2 TUNA MELTS)

Total carbs: 11.9 g | Fiber: 3.8 g | Net carbs: 8.1 g | Protein: 38.7 g | Fat: 51 g | Energy: 644 kcal
Macronutrient ratio: Calories from carbs (5%), protein (24%), fat (71%)

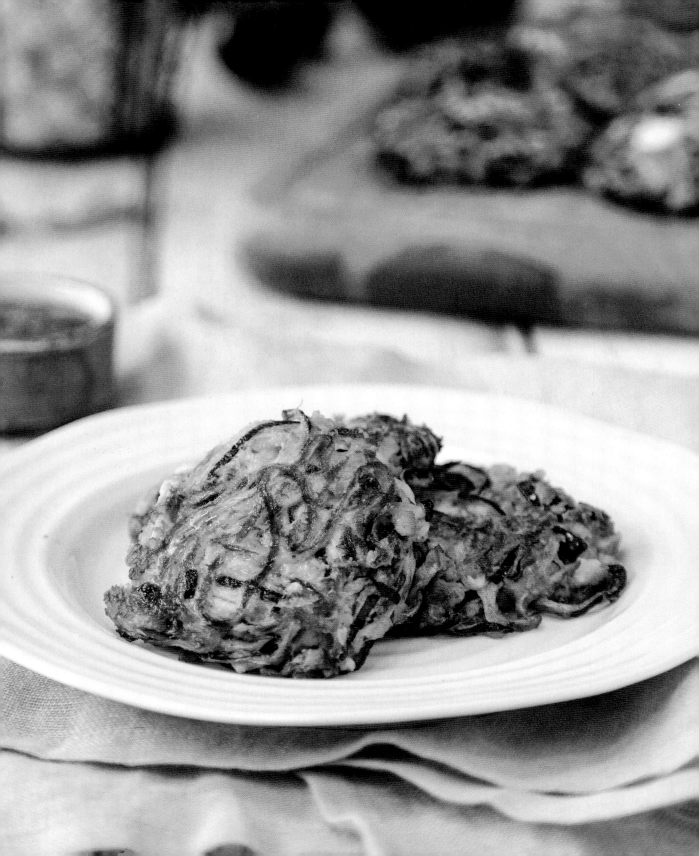

Greek Zucchini and Feta Fritters

These vegetarian fritters are perfect as a light lunch, and they can do double duty as a quick appetizer, too. Try dipping them in full-fat Greek yogurt or Tzatziki (page 159)!

MAKES: 3 SERVINGS (9 PATTIES) | HANDS-ON TIME: 15 MINUTES | OVERALL TIME: 25 MINUTES

2 medium (400 g/14.1 oz) zucchini

½ teaspoon salt, or more to taste

½ cup (45 g/1.6 oz) grated Parmesan cheese

2 large pastured eggs

1 teaspoon ground cumin

½ cup (75 g/2.6 oz) crumbled feta cheese

¼ cup (25 g/0.9 oz) sliced olives

2 tablespoons (8 g/0.3 oz) chopped mixed herbs (such as mint, oregano, and dill)

2 tablespoons (30 g/1.1 oz) ghee or lard

Use a julienne peeler or a spiralizer to create thin "noodles" from the zucchini. Sprinkle them with salt and let sit for 10 minutes. Use a paper towel to pat them dry. (If any noodles are very long, cut them in half.)

Place the zucchini, Parmesan cheese, eggs, cumin, feta, olives, and herbs in a bowl. Combine well. Create small patties from the mixture and fry them in a hot pan greased with the ghee, about 2 to 3 minutes per side. (Do not flip them too early or the patties will break.) Alternatively, you can drizzle the patties with melted ghee and bake them in an oven preheated to 400°F (200°C, or gas mark 6) for 15 to 20 minutes. Once cooked, serve immediately with full-fat yogurt or as a side with meat, or let them cool completely and store in the fridge in an airtight container for up to 3 days.

NUTRITION FACTS PER SERVING (3 FRITTERS)

Total carbs: 7.3 g | Fiber: 2.1 g | Net carbs: 5.2 g | Protein: 15 g | Fat: 25.1 g | Energy: 313 kcal
Macronutrient ratio: Calories from carbs (7%), protein (19%), fat (74%)

CHAPTER 6

Soups and Salads

There's a popular misconception that a low-carb diet is a "no vegetable" diet, but that couldn't be further from the truth. In fact, I make a salad every single day, even if it's just as a side dish. There's no reason to avoid non-starchy vegetables such as broccoli, cauliflower, zucchini, and bell peppers, or fruits like avocado or berries. They're high in micronutrients and low in carbs, and won't impair your weight-loss efforts.

So don't be afraid of fiber-rich foods, and don't get obsessed with carbs or high ketone levels. You don't need to follow a zero-carb diet unless you have a medical condition that requires such an extreme approach. Instead, rejoice in the healthy recipes for comforting, nutritious soups and fresh, easy-to-make salads in this chapter. They're substantial enough to be enjoyed as complete meals.

Beef Ramen

Making a pot of hearty, spicy ramen soup is a great way to use leftover steak—or chicken, or even salmon—from last night's dinner.

MAKES: 4 SERVINGS (ABOUT 8 CUPS/1.9 L/64.8 OZ)
HANDS-ON TIME: 15 MINUTES | OVERALL TIME: 20 MINUTES

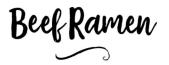

4 medium (60 g/2.1 oz) spring onions

1 tablespoon (6 g/0.2 oz) grated ginger

2 cloves garlic, minced

3 tablespoons (45 g/1.6 oz) ghee or virgin coconut oil, divided

6 cups (1.4 L) beef broth or chicken stock (page 13)

2 tablespoons (30 ml/1 oz) fish sauce

2 tablespoons (30 ml/1 oz) coconut aminos

2 cups (140 g/5 oz) sliced shiitake mushrooms or brown mushrooms

Salt and pepper

2 cups (140 g/5 oz) chopped greens, such as bok choy or collard greens

1 pound (450 g) drained kelp noodles

¼ cup (15 g/0.5 oz) chopped parsley or cilantro, divided

4 large pastured eggs

1 tablespoon (15 g/0.5 oz) Sriracha sauce

¼ cup (60 ml/ 2 oz) extra-virgin olive oil

2 medium (400 g/14.1 oz) steaks, such as sirloin (rump), cooked, cooled, and sliced; or the equivalent amount of salmon or chicken, cooked, cooled, and sliced

Slice the spring onions and separate the green parts from the white parts. Place the white parts of the onions, plus the ginger and garlic, into a medium saucepan greased with 2 tablespoons (30 g/0.5 oz) of the ghee. Cook over medium heat until fragrant. Add the broth, fish sauce, coconut aminos, mushrooms, and salt and pepper to taste. Bring to a boil and add the greens. Cook for 1 to 2 minutes, then remove from the heat. Rinse the kelp noodles and add them to the pot with half of the parsley (reserve the other half for garnish).

To soft-boil the eggs, follow the instructions on page 8 for hard-boiled eggs, leaving them covered in hot water for only 5 to 7 minutes. In a bowl, mix the Sriracha with the olive oil. To assemble, ladle the soup into serving bowls. Add the sliced steak, the green part of the onions, the remaining parsley, and the soft-boiled eggs cut in half. Drizzle the eggs and beef with the spicy oil blend. Serve immediately.

⌒ Instead of zero-carb kelp noodles, which are made from seaweed, you can use shirataki noodles or zucchini noodles (page 8).

NUTRITION FACTS PER SERVING (ABOUT 2 CUPS/480 ML/16.2 OZ)

Total carbs: 8.6 g | Fiber: 2.9 g | Net carbs: 5.7 g | Protein: 34.7 g | Fat: 45.6 g | Energy: 583 kcal
Macronutrient ratio: Calories from carbs (4%), protein (24%), fat (72%)

Cheeseburger Soup

Inspired by everyone's favorite indulgence,
this comforting soup is perfect for cold winter days.

MAKES: 4 SERVINGS (ABOUT 6 CUPS/1.4 L/48.7 OZ)
HANDS-ON TIME: 15 MINUTES | OVERALL TIME: 30 MINUTES

- 1 small (55 g/1.9 oz) white or yellow onion, finely diced
- 1 clove garlic, minced
- 1 tablespoon (15 g/0.5 oz) ghee or lard
- 1 medium (200 g/7.1 oz) rutabaga
- 14.1 ounces (400 g) ground beef
- 2 cups (480 ml/16 oz) bone broth, chicken stock, or vegetable stock (page 13)
- ½ cup (120 g/4.2 oz) unsweetened canned tomatoes
- 1 medium (40 g/1.4 oz) celery stalk, sliced
- ½ cup (70 g/2.5 oz) sliced pickles
- ⅓ cup (75g/2.6 oz) full-fat sour cream
- 1 cup (110 g/3.9 oz) grated Cheddar cheese, divided
- 1 tablespoon (4 g/0.1 oz) chopped parsley, plus more for garnish
- ½ cup (120 ml/4 oz) heavy whipping cream
- 3 pastured egg yolks
- Salt and pepper

Place the onion and garlic in a large soup pot greased with the ghee. Cook over medium heat until fragrant, 3 to 5 minutes. Peel and dice the rutabaga into ½-inch (1 cm) pieces and set aside. Add the beef to the pot and cook for a few minutes until browned on all sides. Pour in the bone broth, add the canned tomatoes, and bring to a boil. Add the rutabaga and celery, and cook for about 5 minutes over medium heat. Add the pickles and cook for another 10 minutes, or until the rutabaga is tender. Add the sour cream. Add the Cheddar cheese, reserving some for topping. Add the parsley and mix well.

Reduce the heat to medium-low. Whisk the cream with the egg yolks in a bowl. (You can use the leftover egg whites to make Candied Spiced Cocoa Pecans [page 180].) Slowly pour the mixture into the soup while stirring. Cook for another minute, then remove from the heat. Season with salt and pepper to taste, top with parsley and the remaining grated Cheddar, and serve.

NUTRITION FACTS PER SERVING (ABOUT 1½ CUPS/360 ML/12.2 OZ)

Total carbs: 10.5 g | Fiber: 2.2 g | Net carbs: 8.3 g | Protein: 30 g | Fat: 54.6 g | Energy: 657 kcal
Macronutrient ratio: Calories from carbs (5%), protein (19%), fat (76%)

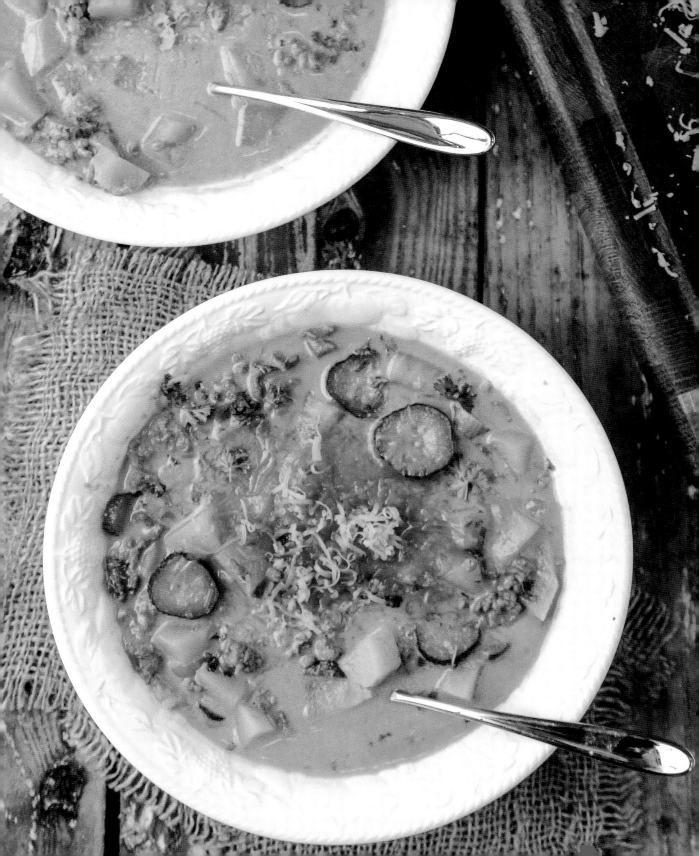

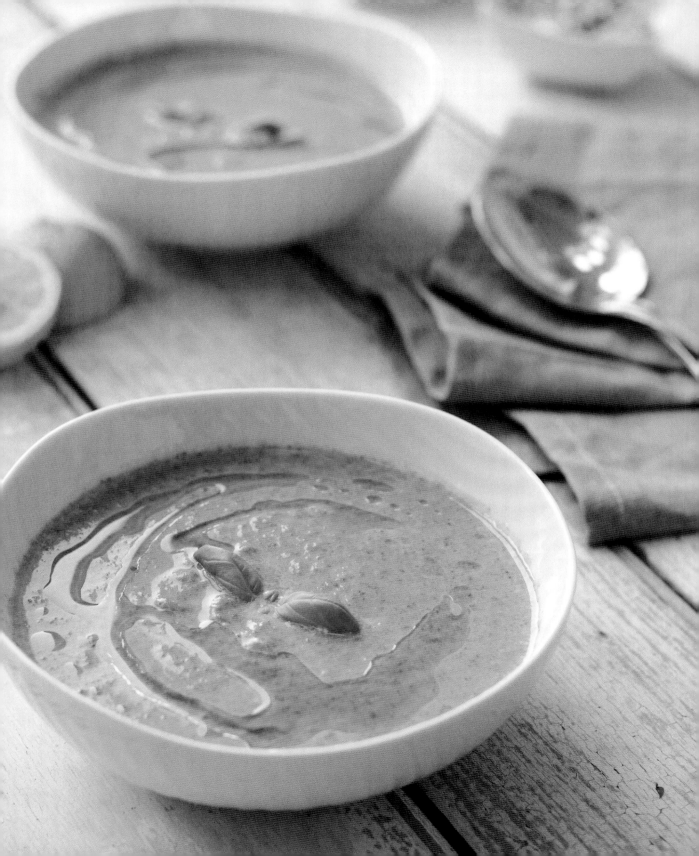

Creamy Broccoli Soup

Don't throw out those leftover broccoli stalks! Use them as an excuse to make this nutritious, creamy soup featuring broccoli, spinach, and blue cheese.

MAKES: 4 SERVINGS (ABOUT 6 CUPS/1.4 L/48.7 OZ)
HANDS-ON TIME: 10 MINUTES | OVERALL TIME: 25 MINUTES

2 tablespoons (30 g/1.1 oz) ghee or lard

1 small (70 g/2.5 oz) white or yellow onion, finely chopped

1 clove garlic, minced

1 small (250 g/8.8 oz) head of broccoli

1 large (64 g/2.3 oz) celery stalk

2 cups (480 ml) chicken stock, bone broth, or vegetable stock (page 13)

7.1 ounces (200 g) fresh or frozen spinach

¼ cup (60 g/2.1 oz) crème fraîche or sour cream

2.6 ounces (75 g) blue cheese, crumbled

1 tablespoon (15 ml/0.5 oz) fresh lemon juice

1 cup (20 g/0.7 oz) fresh basil, plus more for garnish, or 2 tablespoons (30 g/1.1 oz) Avocado and Kale Pesto (page 19)

Salt and pepper

4 tablespoons (60 ml/2 oz) extra-virgin olive oil, divided

Grease a large soup pot with the ghee and heat over medium heat. Add the onion and garlic and cook until fragrant, 3 to 5 minutes. Meanwhile, cut the broccoli into small florets. Peel and dice the broccoli stalk, and slice the celery. Add the broccoli, broccoli stalk, and celery to the pot. Pour in the stock.

Bring to a boil and cook for about 12 minutes. Add the spinach and cook for about 1 minute. Add the crème fraîche, blue cheese, lemon juice, and fresh basil. (Reserve some blue cheese for garnish, if you like.) Remove from the heat and use an immersion blender to process until smooth. (Or, if you're using a regular blender, let the soup cool down slightly before pouring it into the blender.) Taste the soup, add salt and pepper, then pulse again.

Divide among four serving bowls, drizzle each with 1 tablespoon (15 ml/0.5 oz) of the olive oil, and garnish with fresh basil. Serve immediately, or let the soup cool down and store in the fridge for up to 3 days, or freeze in manageable portions for up to 3 months.

NUTRITION FACTS PER SERVING (ABOUT 1½ CUPS/360 ML/12.2 OZ)

Total carbs: 9.6 g | Fiber: 3.4 g | Net carbs: 6.2 g | Protein: 10.6 g | Fat: 34.3 g | Energy: 377 kcal
Macronutrient ratio: Calories from carbs (7%), protein (11%), fat (82%)

Greek Meatball Soup

This soup, known as *youvarlakia avgolemono,* is one of the best soups I've ever made. It's based on my partner Nikos's family recipe, and it only took a couple of small changes to make it keto-friendly.

MAKES: 4 SERVINGS (ABOUT 5 CUPS/1.2 L/40.6 OZ + 12 MEATBALLS)
HANDS-ON TIME: 20 MINUTES | OVERALL TIME: 30 MINUTES

MEATBALLS:

1 tablespoon (15 g/0.5 oz) ghee or lard

1½ cups (180 g/6.3 oz) uncooked cauliflower rice (page 8)

1.1 pounds (500 g) ground lamb or beef

1 large pastured egg

¼ cup (15 g/0.5 oz) chopped parsley, divided

2 tablespoons (8 g/0.3 oz) chopped dill

2 teaspoons (2 g/0.07 oz) onion powder

½ teaspoon ground coriander

½ teaspoon salt

Black pepper

AVGOLEMONO:

4 cups (960 ml/32.5 oz) beef stock or chicken stock (page 13)

3 large pastured eggs

½ cup (120 ml/4 oz) fresh lemon juice (2 to 3 lemons)

¼ cup (60 ml/2 oz) extra-virgin olive oil

To make the meatballs, grease a pan with the ghee and cook the cauliflower rice for 5 to 7 minutes, stirring occasionally. When done, remove from the heat. Place the ground lamb and egg into a bowl. Add the parsley, reserving some for garnish. Add the dill, onion powder, coriander, salt, and pepper. Add the cooked cauliflower rice, and mix until well combined. Shape into 12 medium-size meatballs and set aside.

To make the avgolemono, place the stock in a saucepan and bring to a boil. Turn the heat down to medium-low. Using a slotted spoon, add the meatballs to the boiling stock. Cover with a lid and cook over medium heat for 12 to 15 minutes.

Crack the eggs into a bowl and whisk until frothy. Add the lemon juice and keep whisking. Use a ladle to slowly pour 3 to 4 ladles of the hot stock into the bowl while whisking (in order to bring the egg mix and stock to about the same temperature). Slowly pour the egg and lemon mixture back into the saucepan with the meatballs. Cook for 2 to 3 more minutes over medium heat. Remove from the heat. Just before serving, sprinkle with the reserved parsley and drizzle with the extra-virgin olive oil.

NUTRITION FACTS PER SERVING (ABOUT 1¼ CUP/300 ML/10.1 OZ + 3 MEATBALLS)

Total carbs: 6.6 g | Fiber: 1.4 g | Net carbs: 5.2 g | Protein: 32.6 g | Fat: 51.2 g | Energy: 608 kcal
Macronutrient ratio: Calories from carbs (3%), protein (21%), fat (75%)

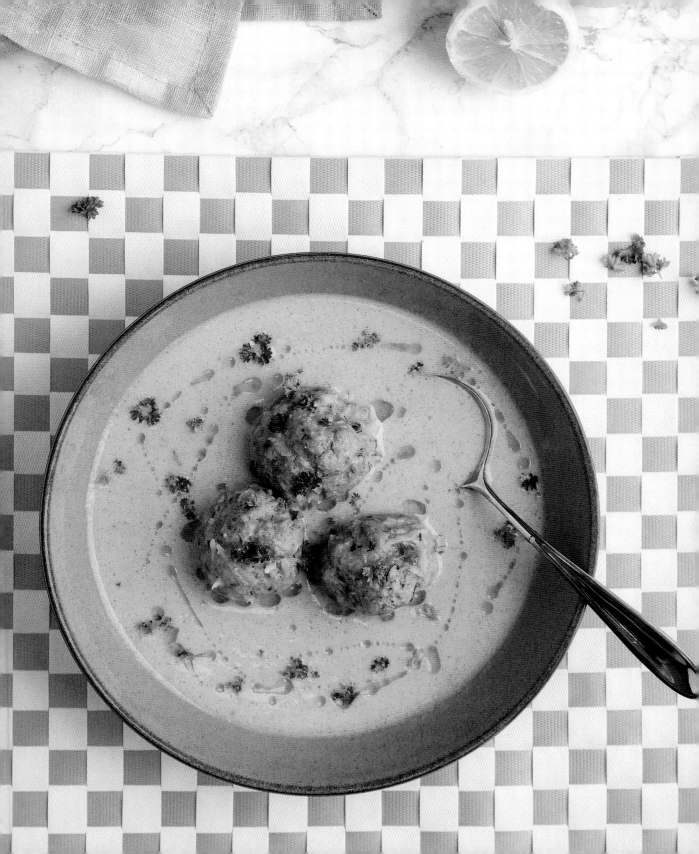

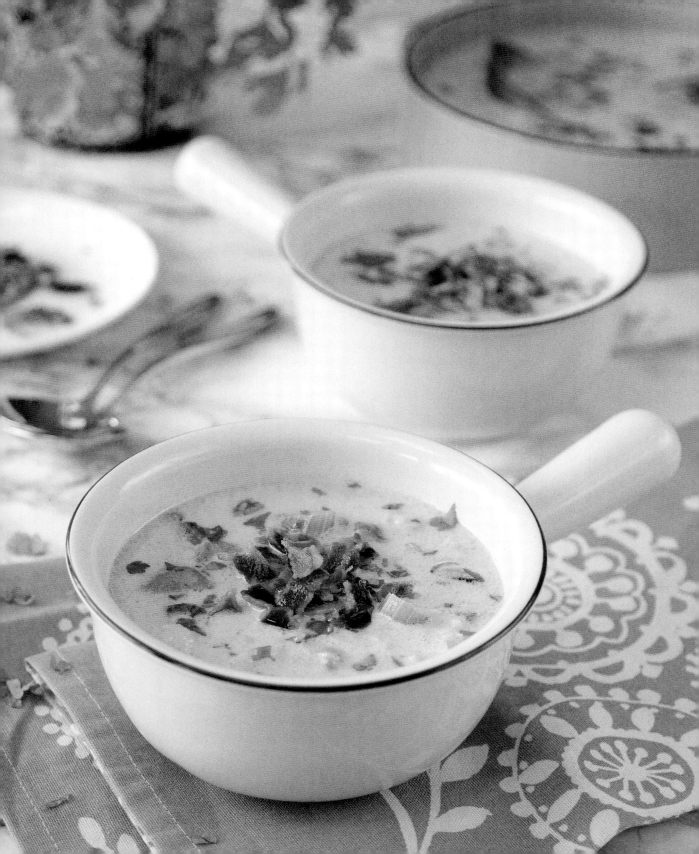

Clam Chowder

This potato-free, flour-free clam chowder is just as good as the traditional version. If you can't find canned clams in a store near you, try canned mussels instead; they work just as well.

MAKES: 6 SERVINGS (ABOUT 7½ CUPS/1.8 L/60.8 OZ)
HANDS-ON TIME: 20 MINUTES | OVERALL TIME: 25 MINUTES

- 1.2 pounds (550 g) chopped clams (or mussels [3 cans, 6.5 oz/182 g each] including the juice)
- ½ medium (300 g/10.6 oz) head cauliflower
- 2 tablespoons (30 g/1.1 oz) ghee or butter
- 1 small (70 g/2.5 oz) white or yellow onion, finely chopped
- 2 cloves garlic, minced
- 2 medium (80 g/2.8 oz) celery stalks, sliced
- 1 cup (240 ml/8 oz) additional clam juice, or chicken stock or vegetable stock (page 13)
- 1 cup (240 ml/8 oz) heavy whipping cream
- 1 cup (230 g/8.1 oz) sour cream
- Salt and pepper
- 2 tablespoons (8 g/0.3 oz) chopped fresh parsley, divided
- 3 large slices (48 g/1.7 oz) crispy bacon for topping (page 10)

Drain the clams and reserve the clam juice. Set aside. Cut the cauliflower into 1-inch florets. Heat a large soup pot or a Dutch oven greased with the ghee over medium-high heat. Add the onion and garlic. Cook until fragrant, 2 to 3 minutes. Add the celery and cauliflower, and sauté for 1 minute.

Pour in the reserved clam juice, additional clam juice or stock. Bring to a boil, then cover with a lid, and reduce the heat to medium. Cook for 5 to 8 minutes, or until the cauliflower is tender. Add the cream, sour cream, and clams, mix well, and heat through for 3 to 5 minutes. Season with salt and pepper to taste. Mix in half the chopped parsley. Serve topped with the remaining parsley and the crispy bacon pieces.

⌒ To make the soup extra-thick, try mixing 4 to 6 egg yolks into the 1 cup (240 ml/8 oz) of cream.

NUTRITION FACTS PER SERVING (ABOUT 1¼ CUPS/300 ML/10.1 OZ)

Total carbs: 9.7 g | Fiber: 1.5 g | Net carbs: 8.2 g | Protein: 19.5 g | Fat: 30.4 g | Energy: 392 kcal
Macronutrient ratio: Calories from carbs (9%), protein (20%), fat (71%)

BLT Deviled Egg Salad

Topped with a creamy, garlicky dressing, this lunchbox-friendly salad is the perfect combination of protein-packed deviled eggs and everyone's favorite sandwich—the classic BLT.

MAKES: 2 SERVINGS | HANDS-ON TIME: 10 MINUTES | OVERALL TIME: 10 MINUTES

DEVILED EGGS:

4 large eggs

2 tablespoons (30 g/1.1 oz) Mayonnaise (page 20)

1 tablespoon (15 ml/0.5 oz) fresh lemon juice or pickle relish

½ teaspoon Dijon mustard

Salt and pepper

DRESSING:

1 clove garlic, crushed

2 tablespoons (30 ml/1 oz) heavy whipping cream or coconut milk

2 tablespoons (30 g/1.1 oz) Mayonnaise (page 20)

Salt and pepper

SALAD:

1 small (200 g/7.1 oz) head crispy lettuce

2 cups (60 g/2.1 oz) salad greens, such as spinach or lamb's lettuce

8 ounces (225 g) cherry tomatoes, halved (or regular tomatoes, chopped)

4 large slices (64 g/2.3 oz) crispy bacon (page 10), cut into 1-inch (2.5 cm) squares

To make the deviled eggs, hard-boil the eggs by following the instructions on page 8.

Meanwhile, to make the salad dressing, mix the garlic, cream, mayonnaise, and salt and pepper to taste in a small bowl.

Assemble the deviled eggs. Cut the eggs in half and carefully—without breaking the egg whites—spoon the egg yolks into a bowl. Add the mayonnaise, lemon juice, and Dijon mustard. Mix using a fork. Season with salt and pepper to taste. Use a spoon to fill in the egg white halves with the egg yolk mixture and set aside.

To assemble the salad, place the lettuce and salad greens into a serving bowl, and top with the tomatoes, bacon, and deviled eggs. Drizzle with the prepared salad dressing, and serve.

⌒ This recipe makes two servings. To store the second serving, simply keep the greens separate from the remaining ingredients and add them just before serving. (They'll stay fresh and crispy for longer.)

NUTRITION FACTS PER SERVING

Total carbs: 8.5 g | Fiber: 2 g | Net carbs: 6.5 g | Protein: 24.6 g | Fat: 44.1 g | Energy: 527 kcal
Macronutrient ratio: Calories from carbs (5%), protein (19%), fat (76%)

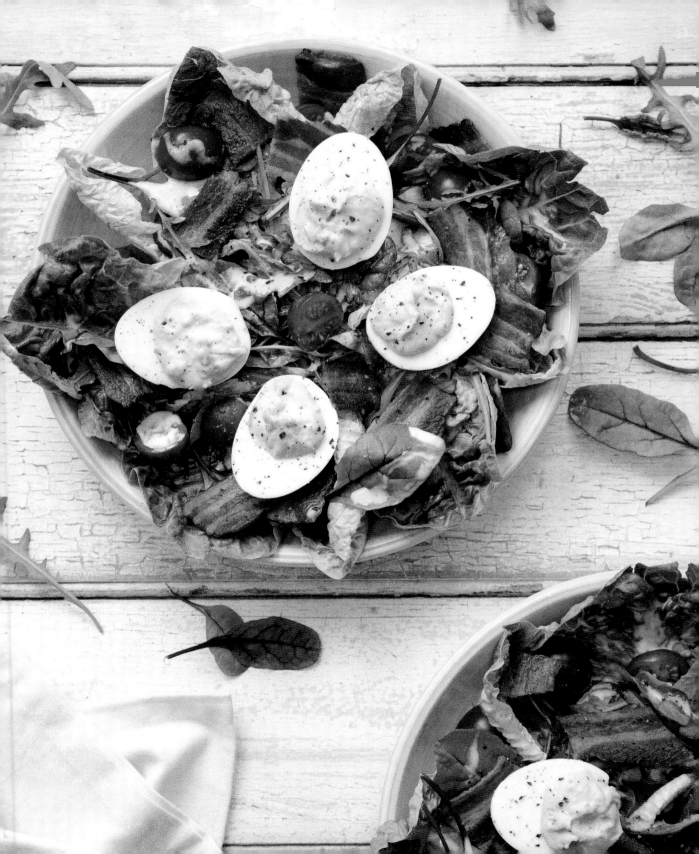

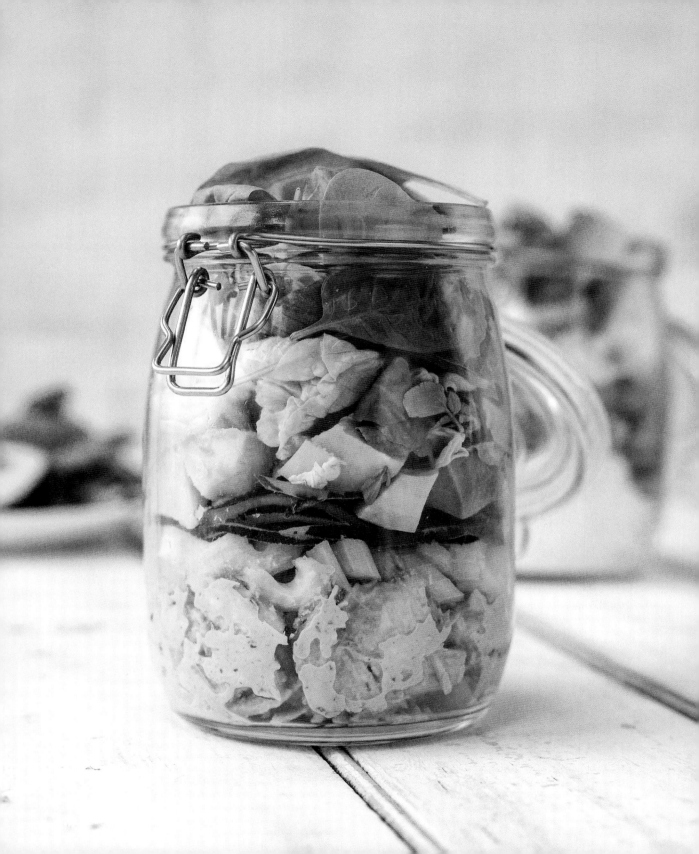

Buffalo Chicken Salad in a Jar

Another great lunchbox option—and an incredibly satisfying one at that!
Plus, it takes just a few minutes to prepare. Use leftover chicken
from last night's dinner; that way, nothing goes to waste.

MAKES: 2 SERVINGS | HANDS-ON TIME: 10 MINUTES | OVERALL TIME: 10 MINUTES

BUFFALO DRESSING:

¼ cup (55 g/1.9 oz) Mayonnaise
(page 20)

3 tablespoons (45 g/1.6 oz)
Sriracha sauce, or to taste

¼ teaspoon paprika

¼ teaspoon garlic powder

¼ teaspoon onion powder

Salt and pepper

2 cups (280 g/9.9 oz) diced
cooked chicken

SALAD:

1 medium (150 g/5.3 oz) avocado

1 tablespoon (15 ml/0.5 oz) fresh
lemon juice

Optional: ⅓ cup (45 g/1.6 oz)
crumbled blue cheese

2 medium (80 g/2.8 oz) celery stalks,
sliced

1 small (60 g/2.1 oz) red onion, sliced

4 cups (120 g/4.2 oz) mixed
salad greens

To make the dressing, add all of the dressing ingredients to a bowl. Mix until well combined, then add the cooked chicken and mix again.

To make the salad, halve, peel, and dice the avocado. Squeeze the lemon juice over the avocado to prevent it from browning. To assemble the salad, divide the dressed chicken between two 1-quart (950 ml) jars with wide mouths. Add a layer of blue cheese (if using) to each jar, followed by the celery, red onion, diced avocado, and salad greens. When ready to serve, tip the salad over into a serving bowl so that the dressing covers the greens. Or, simply shake the jar—keeping the lid closed—and then eat the salad right from the jar. Store sealed in the fridge for up to 3 days.

NUTRITION FACTS PER SERVING

Total carbs: 15.1 g | Fiber: 7.4 g | Net carbs: 7.7 g | Protein: 44.5 g | Fat: 39.7 g | Energy: 589 kcal
Macronutrient ratio: Calories from carbs (5%), protein (32%), fat (63%)

Ranch Salad in a Jar

Packing salads in jars isn't just a passing trend: it's an ingenious way to prepare healthy low-carb meals in advance. This delicious Ranch Salad, for instance, will stay fresh for several days in the fridge.

MAKES: 2 SERVINGS | HANDS-ON TIME: 10 MINUTES | OVERALL TIME: 10 MINUTES

DRESSING:

¼ cup (55 g/1.9 oz) Mayonnaise (page 20)

¼ cup (58 g/2 oz) sour cream

1 tablespoon (15 ml/0.5 oz) apple cider vinegar or fresh lemon juice

¼ teaspoon onion powder

¼ teaspoon garlic powder

⅛ teaspoon paprika

1 to 2 tablespoons (4 to 8 g/0.1 to 0.3 oz) chopped dill

Salt and pepper

SALAD:

2 medium (80 g/2.8 oz) celery stalks, sliced

4 large eggs, hard-boiled (page 8), quartered

4 large slices (64 g/2.3 oz) crispy bacon (page 10), chopped

4 cups (120 g/4.2 oz) mixed salad greens

To make the ranch dressing, combine the mayonnaise, sour cream, vinegar, onion powder, garlic powder, paprika, dill, salt, and pepper. Place the dressing at the bottom of two 1-quart (950 ml) jars with wide mouths. To assemble the salad, add a layer of celery to each jar, followed by a layer of the quartered eggs, then the bacon pieces and salad greens. When ready to serve, tip the salad over into a serving bowl so that the dressing covers the greens. Or, simply shake the jar—keeping the lid closed—and then eat the salad right from the jar. Store sealed in the fridge for up to 3 days.

When you're making salads in jars, be sure to put the dressing at the bottom, followed by a layer of sturdy low-carb vegetables, such as celery, cucumber, or peppers. Add a layer of protein, like eggs or meat. Finally, top with leafy greens. This style of layering will prevent the tender greens from wilting, and they'll stay fresh for longer. Use a wide-mouth jar for easy assembly—and to make it easy to decant the salad into a bowl.

NUTRITION FACTS PER SERVING

Total carbs: 5.1 g | Fiber: 1.5 g | Net carbs: 3.6 g | Protein: 24.3 g | Fat: 41.4 g | Energy: 489 kcal
Macronutrient ratio: Calories from carbs (3%), protein (20%), fat (77%)

Salmon Niçoise

Love niçoise salad? Me, too. Make yours keto-friendly by skipping the potatoes. And, for an extra dose of healthy omega-3s, substitute salmon for the traditional tuna.

MAKES: 2 SERVINGS | HANDS-ON TIME: 15 MINUTES | OVERALL TIME: 25 MINUTES

SALAD:

1½ cups (150 g/5.3 oz) raw green beans, trimmed

1 tablespoon (15 g/0.5 oz) ghee or virgin coconut oil

2 medium (250 g/8.8 oz) salmon fillets

Salt and pepper

2 large eggs

4 cups (120 g/4.2 oz) mixed salad greens

2 small (80 g/2.8 oz) tomatoes, sliced

½ medium (100 g/3.5 oz) cucumber, sliced

½ medium (40 g/1.4 oz) red onion, sliced

8 olives, pitted (24 g/0.8 oz)

4 canned (16 g/0.6 oz) anchovies, chopped, or 2 tablespoons (17 g/ 0.6 oz) capers

DRESSING:

3 tablespoons (45 ml/1.5 oz) extra-virgin olive oil

1 tablespoon (15 ml/0.5 oz) fresh lemon juice

1 clove garlic, crushed

½ teaspoon Dijon mustard

Pinch of salt and pepper

To make the salad, fill a saucepan with salted water and bring to a boil. Add the green beans and cook for 2 to 4 minutes, until they are just al dente. Using a slotted spoon, plunge them into a bowl of ice water to stop the cooking. Transfer them to paper towels to dry.

Grease a pan with the ghee and place over medium-high heat. Pat the salmon fillets dry with paper towels, and season with salt and pepper. Place the salmon, skin-side down, on the hot pan, and lower the heat to medium. Cook for 3 to 4 minutes per side, until the fish is firm and cooked through. (Do not force the fish out of the pan. If you try to flip the fillet and it doesn't release, give it a few more seconds until it becomes crisp, then try again.) Set the cooked fish aside.

To hard-boil the eggs, follow the instructions on page 8: for a soft-set egg yolk, leave covered for 8 to 9 minutes; for a hard-boiled one, up to 13 minutes. When done, peel and cut the eggs into quarters.

Prepare the dressing by combining all the ingredients in a small bowl.

To assemble the salad, place the salad greens into serving bowls. Add the tomatoes, cucumber, onion, and cooked green beans. Top with the salmon fillets (with or without the skin), quartered eggs, olives, and anchovies. Drizzle with the prepared dressing and serve.

NUTRITION FACTS PER SERVING

Total carbs: 12.5 g | Fiber: 4.3 g | Net carbs: 8.2 g | Protein: 39.1 g | Fat: 44.4 g | Energy: 605 kcal
Macronutrient ratio: Calories from carbs (6%), protein (26%), fat (68%)

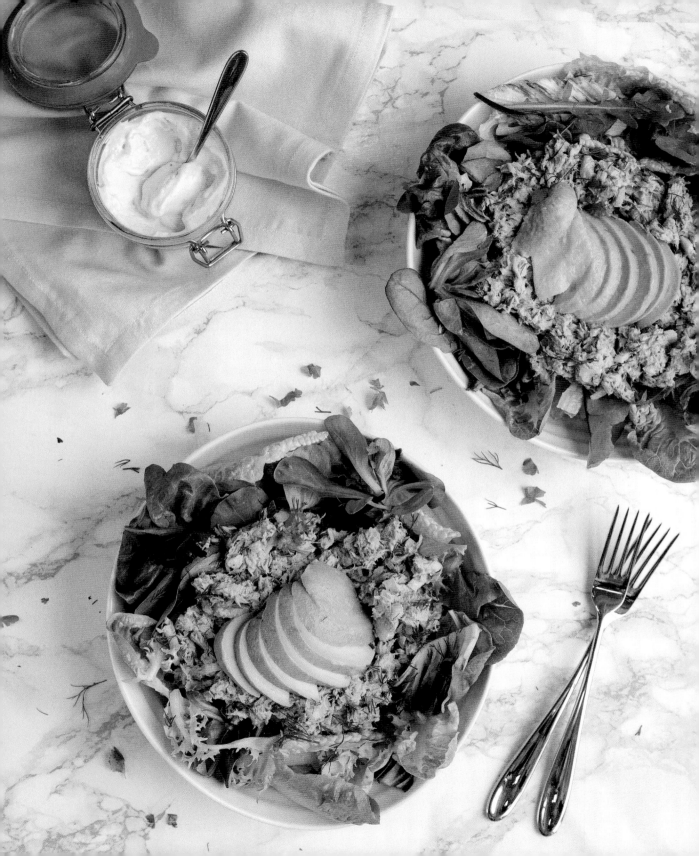

5-Minute Tuna Salad

This is the ultimate quick-prep salad. It literally takes five minutes to toss together. Use any type of canned fish—such as tuna, salmon, mackerel, or sardines—or replace the fish with cooked chicken. And feel free to tweak this salad to taste. For instance, sometimes I skip the celery and top with a hard-boiled egg.

MAKES: 2 SERVINGS | HANDS-ON TIME: 5 MINUTES | OVERALL TIME: 5 MINUTES

1 large can (315 g/12.5 oz) tuna, drained

⅓ cup (75 g/2.6 oz) Mayonnaise (page 20)

2 tablespoons (30 ml/1 oz) fresh lemon juice

1 teaspoon Dijon mustard

1 small (50 g/1.8 oz) white onion, diced

2 cloves garlic, crushed

1 tablespoon (4 g/0.1 oz) chopped fresh parsley, plus more for garnish

1 medium (40 g/1.4 oz) celery stalk, sliced

Salt and pepper

4 cups (120 g/4.2 oz) mixed salad greens

1 medium (150 g/5.3 oz) avocado, peeled, pitted, and sliced

In a bowl, combine the tuna, mayonnaise, lemon juice, Dijon mustard, onion, garlic, parsley, celery, and salt and pepper to taste. Place the salad greens in a serving bowl and add the tuna mixture. Top with the avocado, garnish with more parsley, and serve.

⌒ This recipe works well with other types of fish. Try salmon with lemon juice and chopped dill, or sardines with ½ teaspoon turmeric powder.

NUTRITION FACTS PER SERVING

Total carbs: 12.3 g | Fiber: 6.7 g | Net carbs: 5.6 g | Protein: 34 g | Fat: 43.3 g | Energy: 555 kcal
Macronutrient ratio: Calories from carbs (4%), protein (25%), fat (71%)

Warm Brussels Sprout Salad

Brussels sprouts and slow-cooked meat were made for each other, and this simple, four-ingredient salad is proof. Feel free to experiment with it, though. You can use beef, chicken, or lamb in place of the pork, or shredded cabbage or kale in place of the Brussels sprouts.

MAKES: 4 SERVINGS | HANDS-ON TIME: 10 MINUTES | OVERALL TIME: 25 MINUTES

1.3 pounds (600 g) Brussels sprouts

2 tablespoons (30 g/1.1 oz) ghee or lard, melted

Salt and pepper

1.3 pounds (600 g) Pork Carnitas (page 27) or any type of shredded pork

2 to 4 tablespoons (28 to 60 ml/0.9 to 2 oz) reserved cooking juices, or bone broth or chicken stock (page 13)

Optional: Sriracha sauce

Preheat the oven to 400°F (200°C, or gas mark 6). Wash the Brussels sprouts, pat dry, and slice thinly with a knife (or use a slicing blade on your food processor). Spread the shredded sprouts on a large baking sheet and drizzle with the melted ghee. Season with salt and pepper to taste, then bake for 10 minutes. Remove from the oven. Add the pork and reserved cooking juices to the baking sheet, mixing it with the shredded sprouts. Return the mixture to the oven and bake for another 10 minutes, until the sprouts are soft and the pork is slightly crispy. Let the salad sit for 5 minutes before serving—with a drizzle of Sriracha sauce, if you like.

NUTRITION FACTS PER SERVING

Total carbs: 15.6 g | Fiber: 5.8 g | Net carbs: 9.8 g | Protein: 39.1 g | Fat: 44 g | Energy: 612 kcal
Macronutrient ratio: Calories from carbs (7%), protein (26%), fat (67%)

Caprese Stuffed Avocado

If you read my blog, you'll know that I absolutely love stuffed avocados. They're so nutritious, and so quick and easy to prepare. You only need to add a few ingredients and lunch is served. This is one of my favorite fillings, but I've tried dozens of them over the years. The options are endless!

MAKES: 1 SERVING | HANDS-ON TIME: 5 MINUTES | OVERALL TIME: 5 MINUTES

2 ounces (56 g) mini mozzarella balls or diced mozzarella

1 tablespoon (15 g/0.5 oz) Avocado and Kale Pesto (page 19)

1 tablespoon (15 ml/0.5 oz) extra-virgin olive oil

Salt and pepper

1 medium (150 g/5.3 oz) avocado, halved, seed removed

½ cup (75 g/2.6 oz) cherry or regular tomatoes, chopped

Fresh basil and freshly ground black pepper

Place the mozzarella in a bowl with the pesto and olive oil. Season with salt and pepper to taste, and mix until completely combined. Leaving a ½-inch (1 cm) layer of avocado along the insides of the skins, scoop the middle of the avocado halves out, cut into small pieces, and add to the bowl with the mozzarella. Add the tomatoes to the bowl and combine. Fill the avocado halves with the mixture. Garnish with the fresh basil and black pepper, and enjoy!

NUTRITION FACTS PER SERVING

Total carbs: 17.9 g | Fiber: 11.7 g
Net carbs: 6.2 g | Protein: 18 g
Fat: 50.5 g | Energy: 573 kcal
Macronutrient ratio: Calories from carbs (5%), protein (13%), fat (82%)

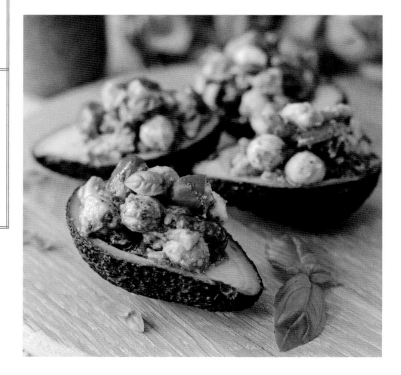

Prawn Cocktail Stuffed Avocado

This meal features a British take on shrimp cocktail with a spicy and creamy sauce (not tomato-based). And it checks all the boxes: It's quick and easy to prepare. It calls for just a few ingredients, and it's high in heart-healthy monounsaturated fats.

MAKES: 1 SERVING | HANDS-ON TIME: 5 MINUTES | OVERALL TIME: 5 MINUTES

3.5 ounces (100 g) cooked shrimp, chopped

2 tablespoons (30 g/1.1 oz) Mayonnaise (page 20)

1 teaspoon Sriracha sauce

1 teaspoon fresh lemon or lime juice

Salt

1 medium (150 g/5.3 oz) avocado, halved, pit removed

Chopped fresh chives, pinch of paprika, and freshly ground black pepper

Combine the shrimp, mayonnaise, Sriracha, lemon juice, and salt in a bowl. Mix until well combined. Leaving a ½-inch (1 cm) layer of avocado along the insides of the skins, scoop the middle of the avocado halves out, and cut into small pieces. Add the avocado to the bowl with the shrimp mixture and stir to combine. Fill the avocado halves with the mixture. Garnish with the chives, paprika, and pepper, and dig in!

NUTRITION FACTS PER SERVING

Total carbs: 15.1 g | Fiber: 10.4 g | Net carbs: 4.7 g | Protein: 23.7 g | Fat: 49 g | Energy: 575 kcal
Macronutrient ratio: Calories from carbs (3%), protein (17%), fat (80%)

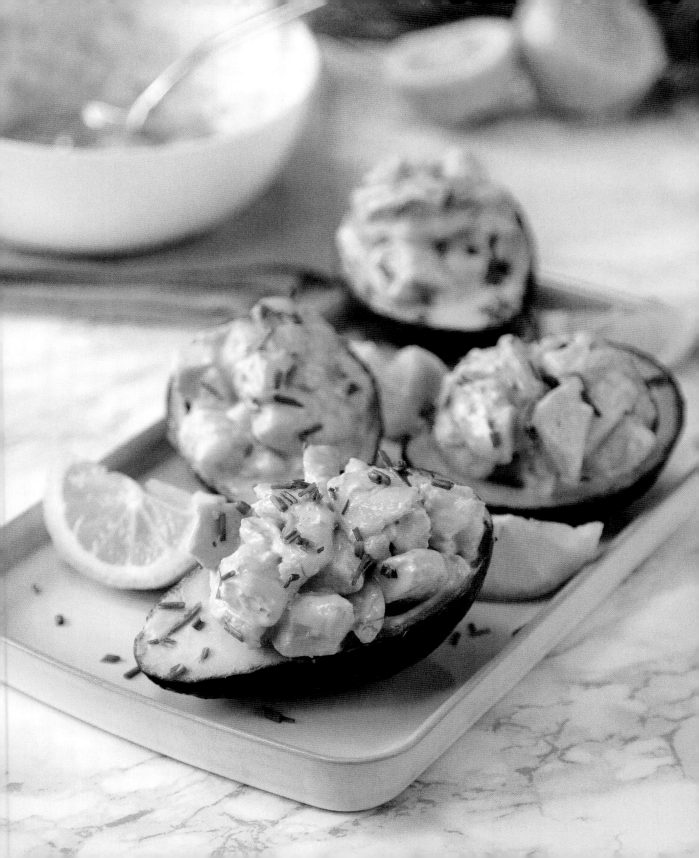

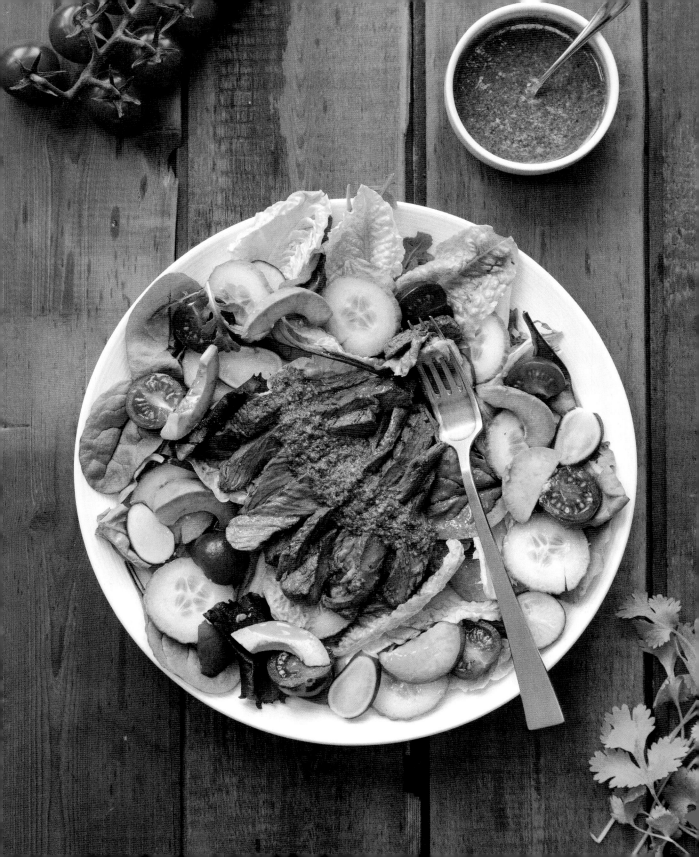

Chimichurri Steak Salad

If you're mourning the loss of those chimichurri steak sandwiches you used to adore, take heart. This salad is every bit as good. I've ditched the bread and added some low-carb veggies, plus an avocado, and the result is both healthy and wonderfully satiating.

MAKES: 2 SERVINGS | HANDS-ON TIME: 15 MINUTES | OVERALL TIME: 20 MINUTES

SALAD:

2 medium (300 g/10.6 oz) rib-eye or sirloin steaks

1 tablespoon (15 g/0.5 oz) ghee or lard

Salt and pepper

4 cups (120 g/4.2 oz) mixed salad greens

½ large (100 g/3.5 oz) avocado, diced

½ medium (100 g/3.5 oz) cucumber, sliced

½ cup (58 g/2 oz) sliced radishes

½ cup (75 g/2.6 oz) cherry or regular tomatoes, sliced

4 tablespoons (60 g/2.1 oz) Chimichurri

CHIMICHURRI:

1 cup (60 g/2.2 oz) chopped parsley, divided

¼ cup (15 g/0.5 oz) chopped fresh oregano, divided

½ cup (120 ml/4 oz) extra-virgin olive oil, divided

4 cloves garlic, sliced

1 small chile pepper, seeded and chopped

2 tablespoons (30 ml/1 oz) red wine vinegar

½ teaspoon salt

¼ teaspoon black pepper

To make the salad, bring the steaks to room temperature by leaving them out on the kitchen counter for 10 to 15 minutes.

Meanwhile, prepare the chimichurri sauce. Place half of each of the parsley, oregano, and oil, plus the garlic, into a blender; set the rest aside. Add the chile pepper, vinegar, salt, and pepper. Pulse until smooth. Add the remaining herbs and oil. Mix until well combined. (Do not pulse again.)

To cook the steaks, grease both sides of the steaks with the ghee and season with salt and pepper. Fry in a hot dry pan over high heat for 2 to 4 minutes on each side to seal in the juices. (When you see the edges start to brown, it's time to flip the steaks over.) Reduce the heat to medium. Continue to cook for another 4 minutes (rare), 7 minutes (medium), or 11 minutes (well done). Remove the steaks from the pan and allow them to rest in a warm place for a few minutes. Slice just before serving.

To assemble, place the salad greens into serving bowls. Add the avocado, cucumber, radishes, and tomatoes. Top each with the sliced steak and chimichurri sauce (about 2 tablespoons [33 g/1.2 oz] per serving). Store any leftover chimichurri in an airtight container in the fridge for up to a week.

⌒ Swap chimichurri with gremolata! To make gremolata, mix ¼ cup (60 ml/2 oz) extra-virgin olive oil with ½ cup (15 g/0.5 oz) parsley, 1 tablespoon (6 g/0.2 oz) lemon zest, 4 cloves minced garlic, ¼ teaspoon salt, and a pinch of black pepper. Serve in place of the chimichurri: use about 2 tablespoons (33 g/1.2 oz) per serving.

NUTRITION FACTS PER SERVING

Total carbs: 11.2 g | Fiber: 6.3 g | Net carbs: 4.9 g | Protein: 31.1 g | Fat: 58.8 g | Energy: 690 kcal
Macronutrient ratio: Calories from carbs (3%), protein (18%), fat (79%)

Quick and Easy Beef Slaw

This spicy, meaty salad is based on "crack slaw," which went viral on the Internet. It is easy to make—maybe even a bit too easy, because it's addictively delicious. Don't say I didn't warn you!

MAKES: 4 SERVINGS | HANDS-ON TIME: 15 MINUTES | OVERALL TIME: 25 MINUTES

2 tablespoons (30 g/1.1 oz) ghee or virgin coconut oil, divided

1.1 pounds (500 g) ground beef

Salt and pepper

1 medium (100 g/3.5 oz) red onion, sliced

2 cloves garlic, minced

1 teaspoon grated fresh ginger

1.3 pounds (600 g) sliced green or white cabbage, or coleslaw mix

1 teaspoon Sriracha or ½ teaspoon red pepper flakes

2 tablespoons (30 ml/1 oz) coconut aminos

1 tablespoon (15 ml/0.5 oz) fresh lemon or lime juice

1 tablespoon (15 ml/0.5 oz) toasted sesame oil

Optional: 1 tablespoon (10 g/0.4 oz) erythritol or Swerve, or 3 to 5 drops liquid stevia extract

Heat a large pan greased with 1 tablespoon (15 g/0.5 oz) of the ghee over medium-high heat. Add the ground beef and cook until browned on all sides. Season with salt and pepper to taste, and use a slotted spoon to transfer to a bowl.

Grease the pan in which you cooked the beef with the remaining 1 tablespoon (15 g/0.5 oz) ghee. Add the red onion, garlic, and ginger. Cook until fragrant and lightly browned, about 3 minutes. Add the cabbage and cook until crisp-tender. Finally, add the Sriracha, coconut aminos, lemon juice, sesame oil, and erythritol (if using). Return the ground beef to the pan and heat through while stirring to allow the flavors to combine. Remove from the heat, and season with salt and pepper to taste. Serve, or let the slaw cool and store in the fridge for up to 3 days, or freeze for up to 3 months.

NUTRITION FACTS PER SERVING

Total carbs: 11.9 g | Fiber: 4.1 g | Net carbs: 7.8 g | Protein: 23.4 g | Fat: 36.2 g | Energy: 462 kcal
Macronutrient ratio: Calories from carbs (7%), protein (21%), fat (72%)

CHAPTER 7:

Dinner

No offense to breakfast, but for most of us dinner is the most important meal of the day. It's probably the only meal you and your family eat together during the workweek, and it might be the only hot meal you have each day. So, being able to quickly whip up tasty, healthy, family-friendly dinners is a big advantage. This chapter will help you do just that. It features dozens of recipes for chicken, fish, beef, lamb, pork, and vegetarian main courses that everyone can enjoy—whether you're following a ketogenic diet or not. Best of all, they require minimal prep, so you won't be spending your entire evening in the kitchen.

Hasselback Chicken

Making Hasselback chicken is just as easy as making Hasselback potatoes (except it's low-carb, of course). You'll slice chicken breasts thinly, then stuff them with ingredients like spices, vegetables, and cheese.

MAKES: 4 SERVINGS | HANDS-ON TIME: 10 MINUTES | OVERALL TIME: 30 MINUTES

CHICKEN:

4 medium (600 g/1.3 lb) chicken breasts

Salt and pepper

4 sun-dried tomatoes (12 g/0.4 oz), chopped, or 2 tablespoons (17 g/0.6) capers, drained

¼ cup (25 g/0.9 oz) sliced olives

¼ cup (60 g/2.1 oz) Avocado and Kale Pesto (page 19)

6 ounces (170 g) regular mozzarella cheese (not fresh or bufala mozzarella)

2 tablespoons (30 ml/1 oz) extra-virgin olive oil

GREEN BEANS:

1.1 pounds (500 g) green beans, trimmed

¼ cup (55 g/1.9 oz) ghee or duck fat, melted

1 tablespoon (15 ml/0.5 oz) lemon juice

Salt and pepper

Preheat the oven to 400°F (200°C, or gas mark 6). To make the chicken, cut 5 to 7 slits widthwise into each breast, about ½ inch (1 cm) apart. Do not slice all the way through the breasts. Season each piece with salt and pepper. Place the sun-dried tomatoes and olives in a bowl and combine with the pesto. Cut the mozzarella into thick slices—as many slices as needed to fill the chicken slits.

Stuff each slit with a slice of mozzarella and a little of the olive-tomato-pesto mixture. (Use about one-quarter of the mixture per chicken breast.) Season the stuffed chicken with salt and pepper, and place on one side of a large baking sheet.

To make the green beans, spread them on the other side of the baking sheet. Drizzle the green beans with the ghee and lemon juice, and season with salt and pepper. Bake for 20 to 25 minutes, until the chicken is cooked through (an instant-read thermometer inserted into the thickest part reads 165°F/74°C) and the cheese is bubbling and lightly browned. Drizzle with olive oil and serve immediately, or let cool and store in the fridge for up to 3 days.

NUTRITION FACTS PER SERVING

Total carbs: 12.6 g | Fiber: 4.4 g | Net carbs: 8.2 g | Protein: 46.1 g | Fat: 41 g | Energy: 602 kcal
Macronutrient ratio: Calories from carbs (6%), protein (31%), fat (63%)

Chicken with Lemon and Tarragon Sauce

This easy weeknight meal is still elegant enough to serve to guests—and the only side dish it needs is lightly steamed broccoli. (Hint: Always serve lean meat like chicken with healthy fats, such as mayonnaise, cream, or avocado.)

MAKES: 4 SERVINGS | HANDS-ON TIME: 15 MINUTES | OVERALL TIME: 25 MINUTES

1.3 pounds (600 g) skinless, boneless chicken thighs

2 tablespoons (30 g/1.1 oz) ghee or lard, divided

1 small (70 g/2.5 oz) white or yellow onion, chopped

½ cup (120 ml/4 oz) chicken stock or vegetable stock (page 13)

¼ cup (60 ml/2 oz) fresh lemon juice

1 cup (240 g/8.5 oz) full-fat crème fraîche or sour cream

2 tablespoons (8 g/0.3 oz) chopped tarragon, divided

1.1 pounds (500 g) fresh broccoli florets

Salt and pepper

Pat the chicken thighs dry with a paper towel. Season with salt and pepper, and place on a hot pan greased with 1 tablespoon (15 g/0.5 oz) of the ghee. Cook over medium-high heat for 1 to 2 minutes, then flip them over and cook for 1 to 2 minutes more. Transfer the browned chicken to a plate and set aside.

Grease the same pan with the remaining 1 tablespoon (15 g/0.5 oz) ghee and add the onion. Cook until fragrant and lightly browned, about 5 minutes, stirring occasionally. Return the chicken to the pan and pour in the chicken stock, lemon juice, crème fraîche, and 1 tablespoon (4 g/0.1 oz) of the tarragon. Bring to a boil, cover with a lid, and lower the heat to medium-low. Cook for about 10 minutes, or until tender and cooked through.

Meanwhile, steam or boil the broccoli until crisp-tender, 3 to 4 minutes, or until it reaches the texture you prefer.

Remove the chicken from the heat and add the remaining 1 tablespoon (4 g/0.1 oz) tarragon. Season with salt and pepper to taste. Mix well, then serve with the cooked broccoli. Alternatively, let the chicken mixture cool and store it in the fridge for up to 4 days, or freeze for up to 3 months.

⌒ Replace the broccoli with broccolini, if you like, or with cooked asparagus or green beans.

NUTRITION FACTS PER SERVING

Total carbs: 12.7 g | Fiber: 3.6 g | Net carbs: 9.1 g | Protein: 35.1 g | Fat: 34.6 g | Energy: 496 kcal
Macronutrient ratio: Calories from carbs (7%), protein (29%), fat (64%)

Parmesan-Crusted Chicken Tenders with Zingy Green Slaw

The ultimate kid-friendly meal! This is a healthy take on chicken tenders, served with a refreshing slaw and a creamy homemade dressing that's perfect for dipping.

MAKES: 6 SERVINGS | HANDS-ON TIME: 20 MINUTES | OVERALL TIME: 20 MINUTES

ZINGY GREEN SLAW:

1 small (500 g/1.1 lb) green cabbage

1 medium (300 g/10.6 oz) bulb fennel

4 medium (60 g/2.1 oz) spring onions, sliced

½ cup (110 g/3.9 oz) Mayonnaise (page 20)

¼ cup (60 ml/2 oz) fresh lemon juice

2 tablespoons (30 ml/1 oz) extra-virgin olive oil

¼ cup (15 g/0.5 oz) chopped parsley

Salt and pepper

THOUSAND ISLAND DRESSING:

½ cup (110 g/3.9 oz) Mayonnaise (page 20)

¼ cup (60 g/2.1 oz) sugar-free ketchup

1 tablespoon (15 g/0.5 oz) Sriracha

1 clove garlic, minced

2 tablespoons (30 ml/1 oz) fresh lemon juice

1 teaspoon onion powder, or 1 small (70 g/7.5 oz) white onion, minced

Salt and pepper

CHICKEN TENDERS:

2 pounds (900 g) skinless, boneless chicken breasts

2 cups (180 g/6.3 oz) grated Parmesan cheese

2 tablespoons (30 g/1.1 oz) ghee or duck fat for frying

To make the slaw, using your food processor's slicing blade, thinly slice the cabbage and fennel, then place in a large mixing bowl. Add the spring onions, mayonnaise, lemon juice, olive oil, and parsley. Season with salt and pepper to taste, and mix well.

To make the dressing, mix all the ingredients in a bowl.

To make the chicken tenders, slice the chicken breasts into strips about ½-inch (1 cm) thick. Place in a bowl with the grated Parmesan and roll to coat well. Heat a pan greased with the ghee over medium-high heat. Once hot, add the chicken tenders, and fry until golden brown on both sides. Work in batches: do not overfill the pan. Use a rubber spatula to flip the chicken halfway through cooking, keeping as much of the Parmesan crust as possible on the tenders. (Alternatively, preheat the oven to 400°F [200°C, or gas mark 6] and bake the Parmesan-coated chicken tenders for 20 to 25 minutes.) Serve the chicken tenders with the slaw and the prepared dressing on the side.

NUTRITION FACTS PER SERVING

Total carbs: 13 g | Fiber: 4.4 g | Net carbs: 8.6 g | Protein: 45 g
Fat: 47 g | Energy: 647 kcal
Macronutrient ratio: Calories from carbs (6%), protein (28%), fat (66%)

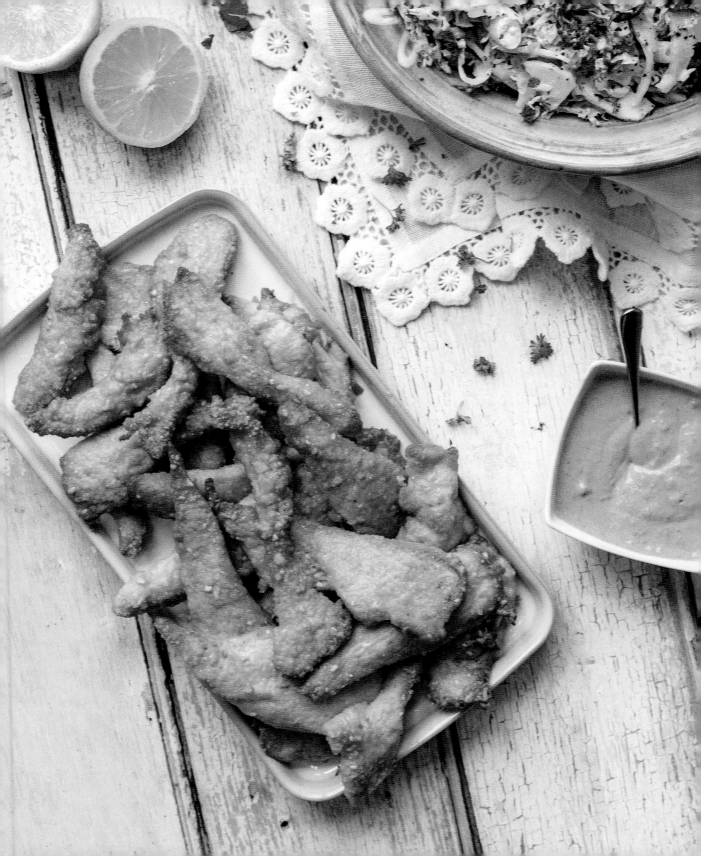

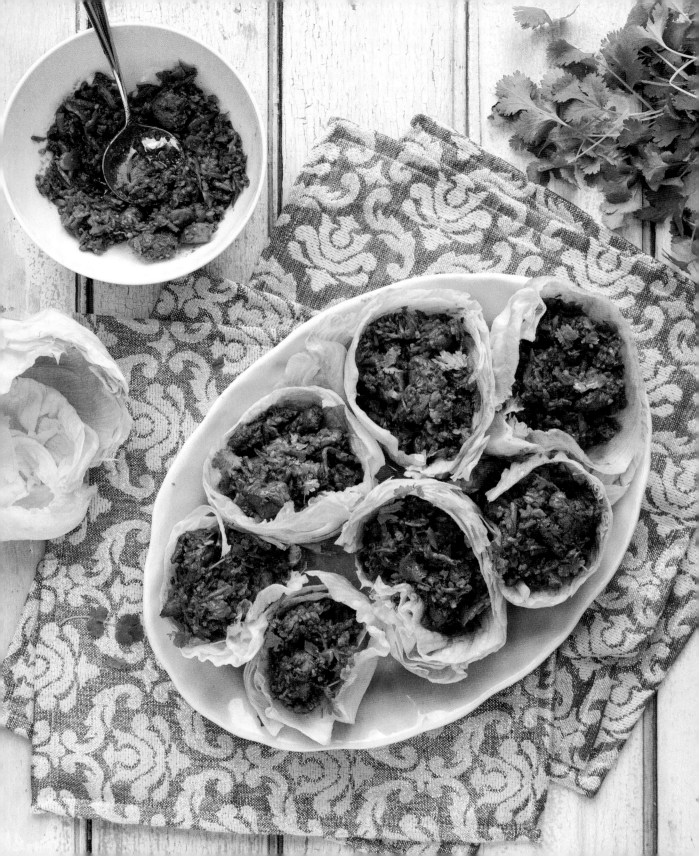

Harissa Chicken Cauli-Cups

Redolent of mild chiles and toasted spices, North African harissa paste peps up chicken in a big way. Add some cauli-rice and serve in crisp lettuce cups, and you've got a healthy, well-balanced meal.

MAKES: 4 SERVINGS | HANDS-ON TIME: 20 MINUTES | OVERALL TIME: 25 MINUTES

¼ cup (55 g/1.9 oz) ghee, lard, or duck fat

1.3 pounds (600 g) skinless, boneless chicken thighs, sliced

¼ cup (60 g/2.1 oz) mild harissa paste

4 cups (480 g/16.9 oz) uncooked cauliflower rice (page 8)

Salt

2 tablespoons (8 g/0.3 oz) chopped fresh parsley or cilantro

1 head (400 g/14.1 oz) iceberg lettuce

¼ cup (60 ml/2 oz) extra-virgin olive oil

Heat a large pan greased with the ghee over medium-high heat. Add the chicken and cook for 3 to 5 minutes, stirring frequently. Add the harissa, stir, and cook for another 5 minutes.

Add the cauliflower rice and cook for an additional 7 to 8 minutes, stirring frequently. Season with salt to taste. Remove from the heat and mix in the parsley. Place 2 large or up to 6 small lettuce leaves on a plate. Top with the chicken, drizzle with the olive oil, and serve.

⌒ Be sure to taste your harissa paste before you use it because some products are spicier than others. Then adjust the amount of harissa as necessary. Also, beware of added sugar and vegetable oils in some products: these should be avoided. I always make a batch of my own harissa and freeze it in individual portions in an ice cube tray. You can find my recipe for harissa paste—plus more homemade ingredients such as Dijon mustard, ketchup, and Sriracha— on my blog: www.ketodietapp.com/blog.

NUTRITION FACTS PER SERVING

Total carbs: 12 g | Fiber: 4.8 g | Net carbs: 7.2 g | Protein: 32.8 g | Fat: 35.9 g | Energy: 496 kcal
Macronutrient ratio: Calories from carbs (6%), protein (27%), fat (67%)

Easy Chicken Korma

This Indian dish tastes way more complicated than it actually is.
Serve it with low-carb cauli-rice. You'll never crave takeout again!

MAKES: 4 SERVINGS | HANDS-ON TIME: 15 MINUTES | OVERALL TIME: 30 MINUTES

MEAT SAUCE:

1.3 pounds (600 g) skinless, boneless chicken thighs

¼ cup (55 g/1.9 oz) ghee or virgin coconut oil

1 small (70 g/2.5 oz) onion, chopped

2 cloves garlic, minced

1 tablespoon (6 g/0.2 oz) grated ginger

2 teaspoons (4 g/0.1 oz) each curry powder and garam masala

½ teaspoon each turmeric powder and chili powder

1 cup (240 g/8.5 oz) unsweetened canned tomatoes

Salt and pepper

¼ cup (60 ml/2 oz) creamed coconut milk (page 10) or heavy whipping cream

Optional: 2 heaping tablespoons (16 g/0.6 oz) almond flour, or 2 teaspoons (5 g/0.2 oz) coconut flour

CAULIFLOWER RICE:

2 tablespoons (30 g/1.1 oz) ghee or virgin coconut oil

4 cups (480 g/16.9 oz) cauliflower rice (page 8)

Salt and pepper

Chopped fresh cilantro

To make the meat sauce, dice the chicken into about 1½-inch (4 cm) chunks and set aside. Heat a large saucepan or casserole dish over medium-high heat. Add the ghee, onion, garlic, and ginger. Cook until fragrant, 3 to 5 minutes, stirring constantly. Add the curry powder, garam masala, turmeric powder, and chili powder, stir, and cook for another minute.

Pour in the tomatoes, add the chicken pieces, and stir well until the chicken is covered in the mixture. Season with a pinch of salt and pepper, and bring to a boil. Reduce the heat to medium, cover, and cook for 15 minutes, stirring occasionally. Remove the lid and add the creamed coconut milk. Add the almond or coconut flour (if using); this will make for a thicker sauce. Stir and cook for another 5 minutes. Remove from the heat and set aside.

To make the cauliflower rice, grease a pan with the ghee. Add the cauliflower rice and cook for 5 to 7 minutes, stirring constantly. Season with salt and pepper to taste, and serve with the chicken korma. Garnish with the chopped cilantro.

NUTRITION FACTS PER SERVING

Total carbs: 13 g | Fiber: 4.5 g | Net carbs: 8.5 g | Protein: 32.8 g
Fat: 33.3 g | Energy: 478 kcal
Macronutrient ratio: Calories from carbs (7%), protein (28%), fat (65%)

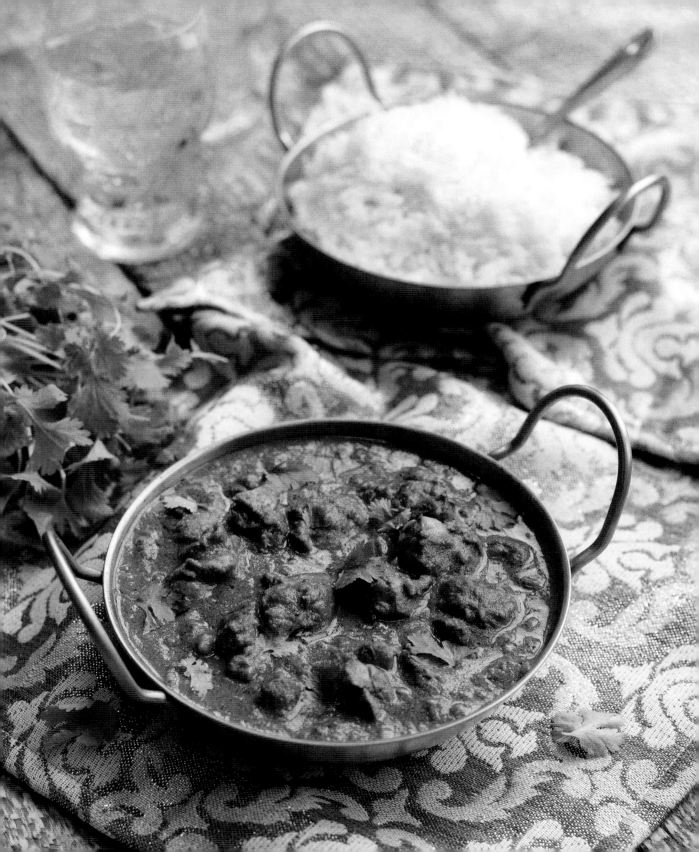

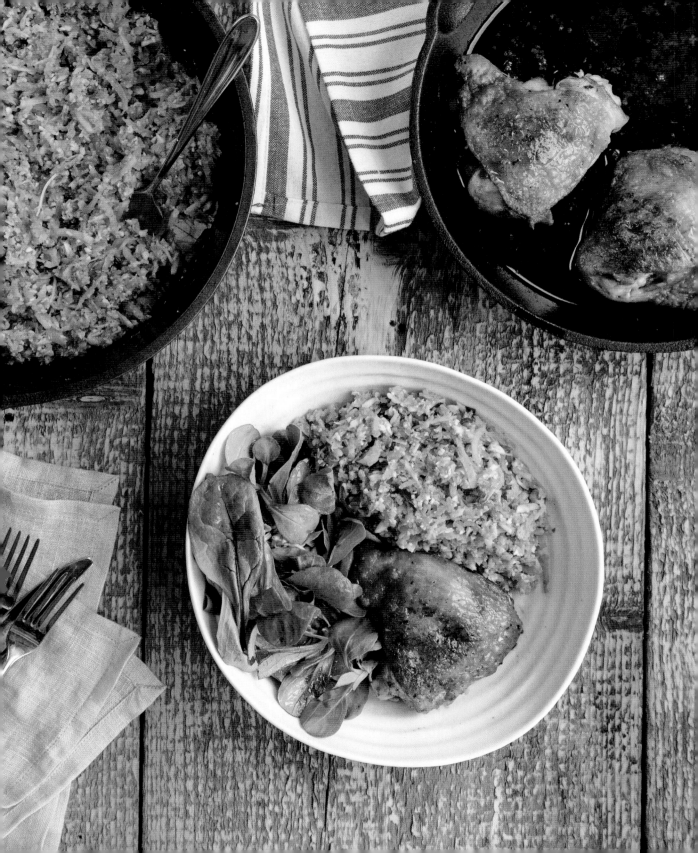

Crispy Skillet Chicken

Crispy on the outside, and wonderfully soft and juicy on the inside, this skillet chicken dish makes an effortless midweek dinner. Serve it with my low-carb version of rice pilaf.

MAKES: 4 SERVINGS | HANDS-ON TIME: 15 MINUTES | OVERALL TIME: 30 MINUTES

CHICKEN:

4 large (800 g/1.76 lb total) chicken thighs, with skin and bone in, or 1.3 pounds (600 g) boneless thighs

1 teaspoon salt

½ teaspoon black pepper

2 tablespoons (30 g/1.1 oz) ghee or duck fat

Optional: ⅓ cup (30 g/1.1 oz) grated Parmesan cheese

RICE PILAF:

¼ cup (55 g/1.9 oz) ghee or duck fat

½ teaspoon onion powder

½ teaspoon garlic powder

½ teaspoon paprika

½ teaspoon ground turmeric

⅛ teaspoon cayenne pepper

6 cups (720 g/1.6 lb) cauliflower rice (page 8)

½ teaspoon salt, or to taste

½ cup (120 ml/4 oz) chicken stock or bone broth (page 13)

2 tablespoons (8 g/0.3 oz) chopped fresh parsley or cilantro

SERVE WITH:

4 cups (120 g/4.2 oz) leafy greens

2 tablespoons (30 ml/1 oz) extra-virgin olive oil

To make the chicken, preheat the oven to 425°F (220°C, or gas mark 7). Pat the chicken thighs dry with a paper towel, then season with the salt and pepper. Heat a large oven-proof pan greased with the ghee. Once hot, add the chicken thighs skin-side down and cook for about 5 minutes, until the skin is golden and crispy. Flip them over and cook for 1 additional minute.

Transfer the thighs, skin-side up, to a wire rack placed inside a baking dish (to help the chicken become crispy during baking). Repeat the pan-frying process for the remaining thighs, then place the baking dish in the oven. Cook for about 15 minutes (for boneless thighs, cook for 10 minutes). If you're using the Parmesan, sprinkle it on top of the thighs for the last 5 minutes of the cooking process.

While the chicken is baking, prepare the rice pilaf. Place the ghee in a large pot and add the onion powder, garlic powder, paprika, turmeric, and cayenne pepper. Add the cauli-rice and cook over medium heat for 2 minutes while stirring. Add the salt. Pour in the chicken stock and cook for another 5 to 7 minutes, stirring occasionally. Remove from the heat and add the parsley. Mix until well combined, and season with more salt and pepper if needed. Serve immediately with leafy greens drizzled with olive oil.

NUTRITION FACTS PER SERVING

Total carbs: 10.6 g | Fiber: 4.3 g | Net carbs: 6.3 g | Protein: 33.6 g | Fat: 35.4 g | Energy: 492 kcal
Macronutrient ratio: Calories from carbs (5%), protein (28%), fat (67%)

Bacon-Rubbed BBQ Chicken Skewers

Now that you know how to make your own Bacon BBQ Sauce (page 30),
why not put it to good use in a batch of fun-to-eat chicken skewers? For best results,
let the meat marinate overnight, or for up to 24 hours, before cooking.

MAKES: 4 SERVINGS | HANDS-ON TIME: 10 MINUTES | OVERALL TIME: 25 MINUTES + MARINATING

CHICKEN:

1.3 pounds (600 g) boneless and skinless chicken thighs

½ cup (120 g/4.2 oz) Bacon BBQ Sauce (page 30)

2 tablespoons (30 ml/1 oz) extra-virgin olive oil

GRILLED ZUCCHINI SALAD:

2 medium (400 g/14.1 oz) zucchini, chopped

2 bunches (300 g/10.6) asparagus

2 medium (30 g/1.1 oz) spring onions, sliced

2 tablespoons (8 g/0.2 oz) chopped fresh mint or parsley, divided

1 tablespoon (15 ml/0.5 oz) fresh lemon juice

2 tablespoons (30 g/1.1 oz) ghee or butter, melted

Salt and pepper

2 tablespoons (30 ml/1 oz) extra-virgin olive oil

To make the chicken, cut the thighs into medium pieces (1 to 1½ inches/3 to 4 cm). Place them in a bowl, and add the Bacon BBQ Sauce and olive oil. Stir to combine. Cover with plastic wrap and refrigerate for 1 to 2 hours (or for up to 24 hours).

When the meat is ready, preheat the broiler to 450°F (230°C, or gas mark 8). Thread the chicken pieces onto skewers and place on a wire rack set inside a baking tray.

To make the zucchini salad, place the zucchini in another baking tray. Add the asparagus, spring onions, and chopped mint. (Reserve some mint for garnish.) Drizzle the vegetables with the lemon juice and melted ghee, and season with salt and pepper.

Place both the chicken skewers and the vegetables in the oven and cook for 12 to 15 minutes. Remove from the oven and let cool for 5 minutes before serving. Garnish the vegetables and skewers with the reserved mint and drizzle with the olive oil.

NUTRITION FACTS PER SERVING

Total carbs: 8.9 g | Fiber: 3.3 g | Net carbs: 5.6 g | Protein: 33.1 g | Fat: 29.2 g | Energy: 428 kcal
Macronutrient ratio: Calories from carbs (5%), protein (32%), fat (63%)

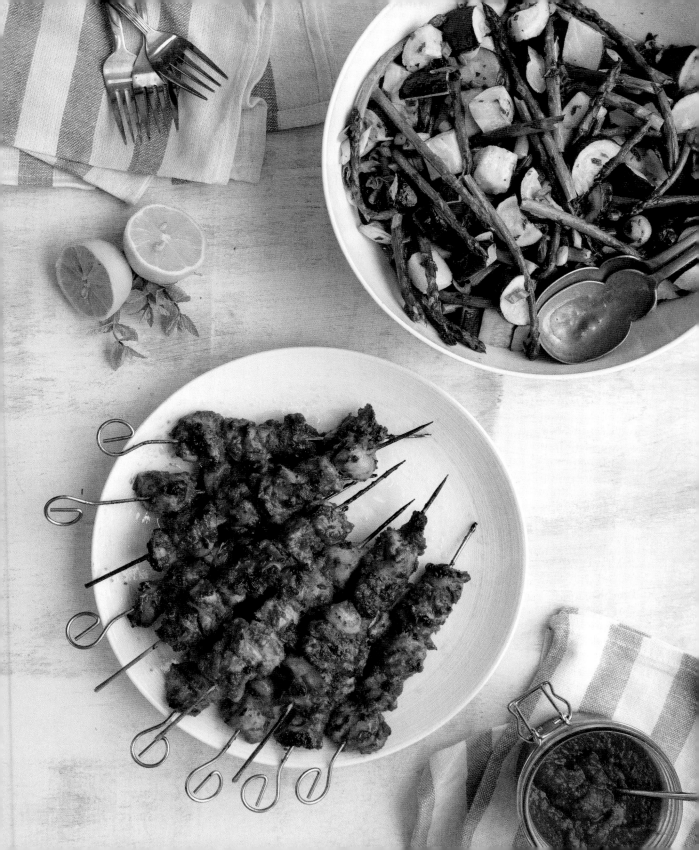

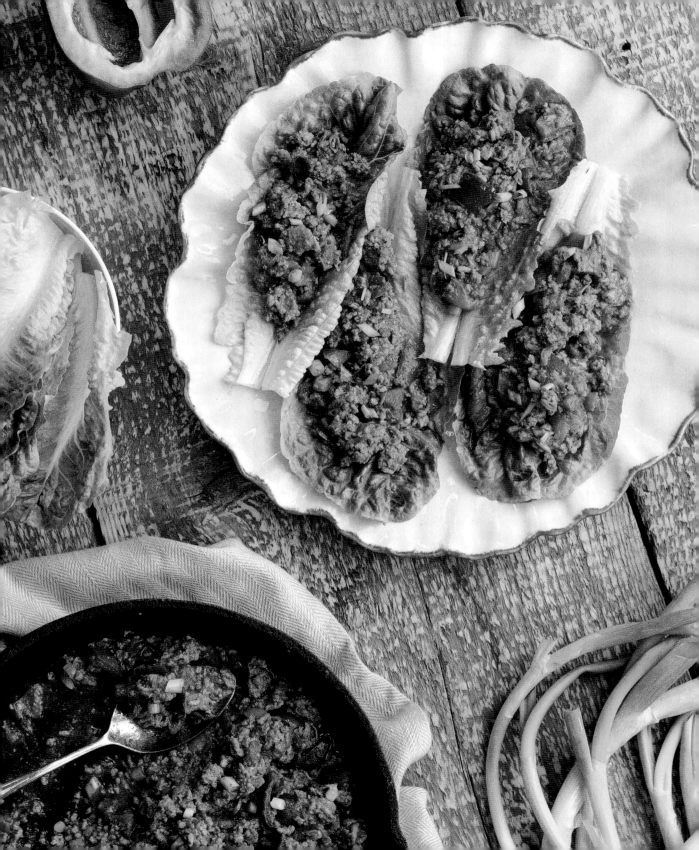

Sloppy Joe Lettuce Cups

Good news for your inner nine-year-old: Sloppy Joes are naturally keto-friendly!
Just be sure to ditch the bun and serve them with romaine or iceberg lettuce instead.

MAKES: 4 SERVINGS | HANDS-ON TIME: 10 MINUTES | OVERALL TIME: 25 MINUTES

2 tablespoons (30 g/1.1 oz) ghee or duck fat

1 small (70 g/2.5 oz) white or yellow onion, chopped

1 large (165 g/5.8 oz) green pepper, sliced

1.1 pounds (500 g) ground turkey

1 teaspoon chili powder

1 teaspoon Dijon mustard

1 tablespoon (15 ml/0.5 oz) apple cider vinegar

¼ cup (60 g/2.1 oz) unsweetened tomato paste

1½ cups (270 g/9.5 oz) chopped fresh or canned tomatoes

Salt and pepper

14.1 ounces (400 g) lettuce (2 medium heads romaine lettuce or 1 head iceberg lettuce)

2 medium (30 g/1.1 oz) spring onions, sliced

¼ cup (60 ml/2 oz) extra-virgin olive oil

Grease a large pan with the ghee and set over a medium-high heat. Once hot, add the onion and green pepper. Cook for 2 to 3 minutes, stirring occasionally. Add the ground turkey, chili powder, Dijon mustard, and vinegar. Cook until the turkey is browned on all sides, 7 to 8 minutes. Add the tomato paste and chopped tomatoes, and bring to a boil. Reduce the heat to medium and cook for 8 to 10 minutes, until thickened. Season with salt and pepper to taste. Remove from the heat and set aside to cool for 5 minutes.

Serve by placing spoonfuls of the mixture on top of lettuce leaves. Sprinkle each with the spring onions and drizzle with the olive oil. Store the Sloppy Joe mixture in an airtight container in the fridge for up to 3 days, or freeze for up to 3 months (without the lettuce).

NUTRITION FACTS PER SERVING

Total carbs: 10.8 g | Fiber: 3.6 g | Net carbs: 7.2 g | Protein: 23.4 g | Fat: 37.5 g | Energy: 462 kcal
Macronutrient ratio: Calories from carbs (6%), protein (20%), fat (74%)

Turkey and Chorizo Sliders with Guacamole

These miniature turkey-chorizo burgers get a Mexican-style kick from guacamole, which is rich in vitamin E, B vitamins, and potassium.

MAKES: 4 SERVINGS (12 SLIDERS) | HANDS-ON TIME: 20 MINUTES | OVERALL TIME: 20 MINUTES

MEAT PATTIES:

14.1 ounces (400 g) ground turkey

7.1 ounces (200 g) Mexican Chorizo (page 26)

½ teaspoon salt

1 tablespoon (15 g/0.5 oz) ghee

GUACAMOLE:

3 large (400 g/14.1 oz) avocados

1 small (70 g/2.5 oz) white or yellow onion, finely chopped

2 cloves garlic, minced

1⅓ cups (200 g/7.1 oz) regular or cherry tomatoes, chopped

1 or 2 small chile peppers, chopped

2 tablespoons (30 ml/1 oz) fresh lime juice, or more to taste

¼ cup (10 g/0.4 oz) chopped fresh cilantro

Salt and pepper

1 head (400 g/14.1 oz) iceberg lettuce

To make the patties, combine the turkey and chorizo in a bowl. Use your hands to shape the mixture into 12 medium patties. Season with salt on both sides. Cook the patties in a hot pan greased with the ghee over medium-high heat for 4 to 5 minutes on each side. Set aside.

To make the guacamole, halve and peel the avocados, remove the seeds, and place half the avocado into a bowl. Mash it well with a fork. Add the onion, garlic, tomatoes, chile pepper, lime juice, and cilantro. Dice the rest of the avocado and mix it into the guacamole, but do not mash it. Season with salt and black pepper to taste.

Tear the lettuce into leaves. Spread the guacamole on top of the lettuce leaves, and serve with the cooked patties. Store the sliders in the fridge—separately from the guacamole—for up to 4 days, or freeze them for up to 3 months. Guacamole can be stored in an airtight container in the fridge for up to 3 days.

NUTRITION FACTS PER SERVING (3 PATTIES + GUACAMOLE AND LETTUCE)

Total carbs: 17.2 g | Fiber: 9.6 g | Net carbs: 7.6 g | Protein: 28.5 g | Fat: 37.4 g | Energy: 501 kcal
Macronutrient ratio: Calories from carbs (6%), protein (24%), fat (70%)

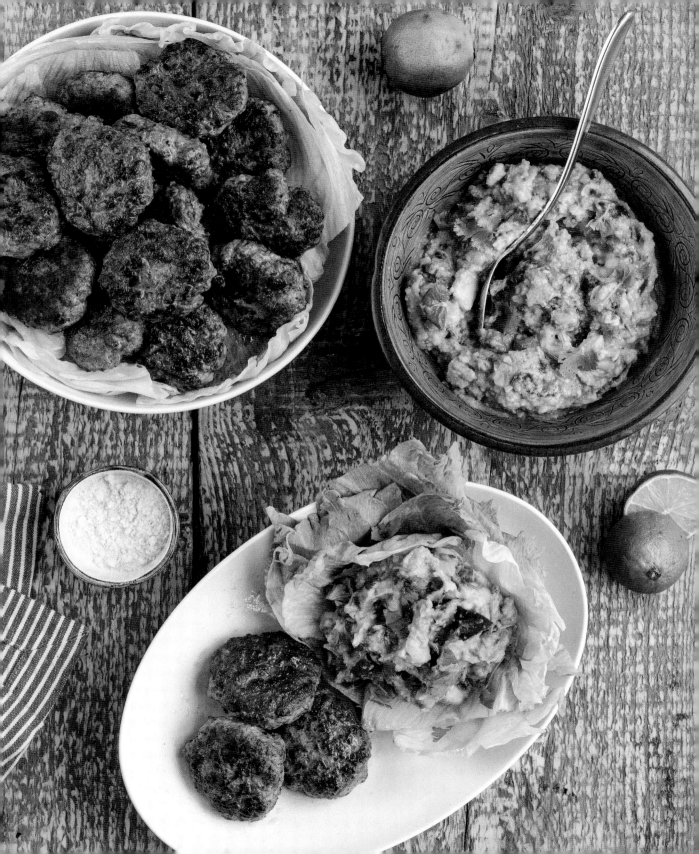

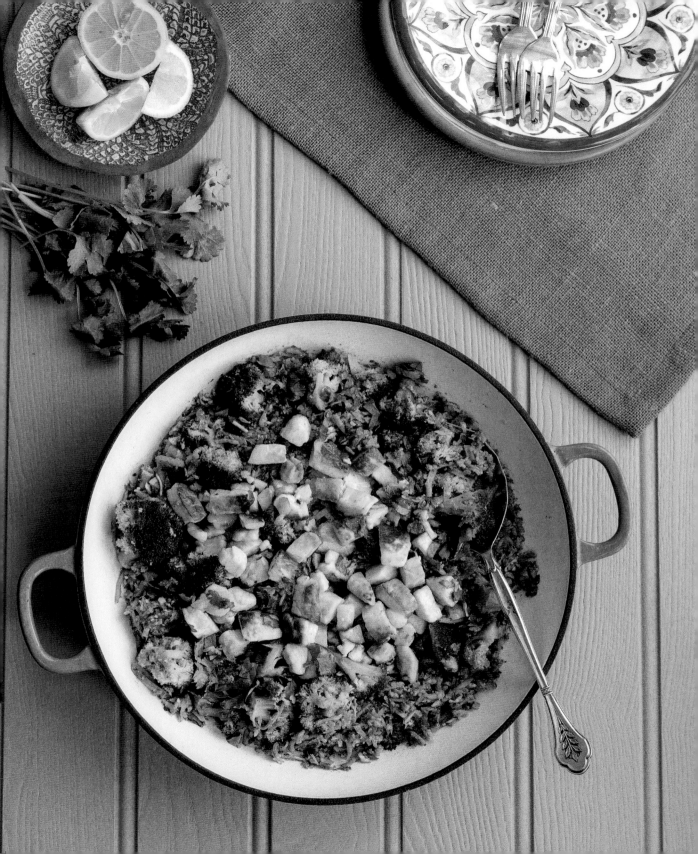

Moroccan Couscous with Halloumi

This vegetarian meal is one of the best ways to enjoy soft, springy Halloumi cheese—paired with plenty of bold flavors and lots of healthy fats.

MAKES: 4 SERVINGS | HANDS-ON TIME: 15 MINUTES | OVERALL TIME: 25 MINUTES

1 package (250 g/8.8 oz) Halloumi cheese

1 small (200 g/7.1 oz) head broccoli

¼ cup (55 g/1.9 oz) ghee or coconut oil, divided

1 small (70 g/2.5 oz) white or yellow onion, chopped

2 cloves garlic, minced

½ teaspoon ground cumin

½ teaspoon ground coriander

¼ teaspoon ground cinnamon

4 cups (480 g/16.9 oz) uncooked cauliflower rice (page 8)

2 tablespoons (30 ml/1 oz) fresh lemon or lime juice

2 to 4 tablespoons (30 to 60 ml/ 1 to 2 oz) water or vegetable stock (page 13)

Salt and pepper

¼ cup (10 g/0.4 oz) chopped fresh cilantro

2 tablespoons (30 ml/1 oz) extra-virgin olive oil

Dice the Halloumi cheese into ½-inch (1 cm) pieces. Cut the broccoli into 1-inch (2 cm) florets. Grease a large pan with 2 tablespoons (27.5 g/0.8 oz) of the ghee and set over medium-high heat. Add the diced Halloumi cheese and cook until crisp, 5 to 8 minutes. Use a slotted spoon to transfer the Halloumi to a bowl. Set aside.

Grease the pan with the remaining 2 tablespoons (27.5 g/0.8 oz) ghee. Add the onion and garlic and cook until fragrant, 3 to 5 minutes. Stir in the cumin, coriander, and cinnamon, followed by the broccoli, cauliflower rice, lemon juice, and water. Season with salt and pepper to taste. Cook until the broccoli is tender, 7 to 8 minutes. (Parboiled broccoli will take less time to cook [page 11].) Add the cooked Halloumi and cilantro. Drizzle the mixture with the olive oil. Serve immediately, or let cool and store in an airtight container in the fridge for up to 5 days.

NUTRITION FACTS PER SERVING

Total carbs: 13.3 g | Fiber: 4.3 g | Net carbs: 9 g | Protein: 16.6 g | Fat: 38 g | Energy: 449 kcal
Macronutrient ratio: Calories from carbs (8%), protein (15%), fat (77%)

Speedy Cauliflower-n-Cheese

This low-carb, cauliflower-based version of mac and cheese is healthier than the original, but it doesn't skimp on taste. A creamy, homemade cheese sauce, c rumbled bacon, and Parmesan cheese make it a hearty, cold-weather treat.

MAKES: 4 SERVINGS | HANDS-ON TIME: 10 MINUTES | OVERALL TIME: 30 MINUTES

CAULIFLOWER BAKE:

1 medium (600 g/1.3 lb) head cauliflower

4 large (64 g/2.3 oz) slices crispy bacon (page 10), crumbled

2 medium (30 g/1.1 oz) spring onions, sliced

⅓ cup (30 g/1.1 oz) grated Parmesan cheese

CHEESE SAUCE:

¼ cup (56 g/2 oz) butter

½ cup (120 ml/4 oz) heavy whipping cream

½ cup (120 g/4.2 oz) cream cheese

½ teaspoon garlic powder

1½ cups (170 g/6 oz) grated Cheddar cheese, divided

To make the cauliflower bake, preheat the oven to 450°F (230°C, or gas mark 8). Cut the cauliflower into 1-inch (2 cm) pieces. Place them in a steamer and cook for 8 to 10 minutes. Once cooked, remove the lid and let the cauliflower cool for 5 minutes.

Meanwhile, prepare the cheese sauce. Place the butter and cream in a small saucepan and heat gently. When hot, add the cream cheese and garlic powder. Stir until melted and bring to a simmer. Once you see bubbles, remove from the heat. Add 1 cup (113 g/4 oz) of the Cheddar cheese, and mix until smooth and creamy.

Place the cooked cauliflower in a baking dish. Add the bacon, spring onions, and prepared cheese sauce. Mix with a spoon until the cauliflower is completely coated, and top with the grated Parmesan and remaining ½ cup (57 g/2 oz) Cheddar cheese. Bake for 10 to 12 minutes, until the top is crispy and golden brown. Remove from the oven and serve immediately, or let it cool and refrigerate for up to 4 days.

NUTRITION FACTS PER SERVING

Total carbs: 10.9 g | Fiber: 3.3 g | Net carbs: 7.6 g | Protein: 23.9 g | Fat: 49.3 g | Energy: 560 kcal
Macronutrient ratio: Calories from carbs (5%), protein (17%), fat (78%)

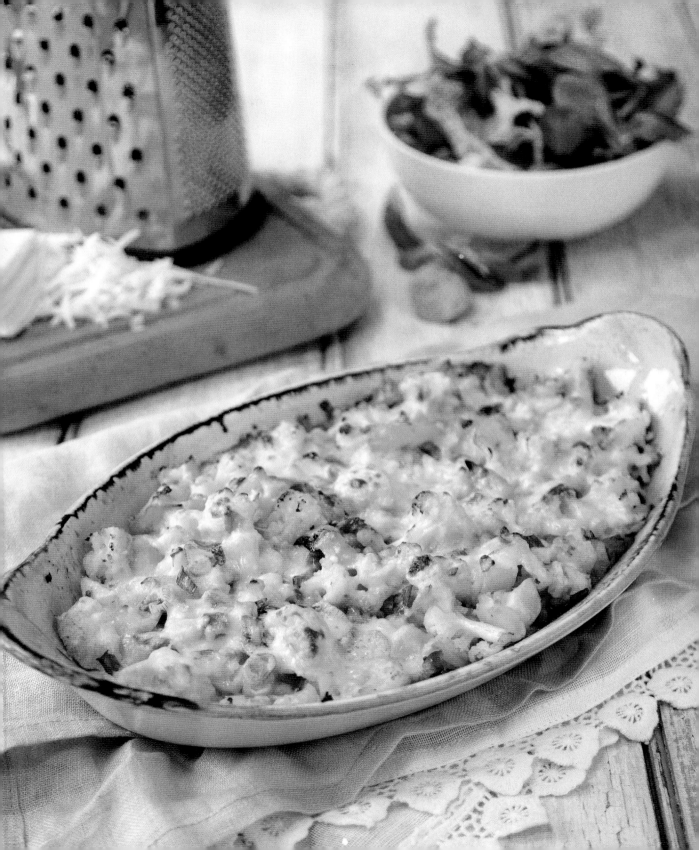

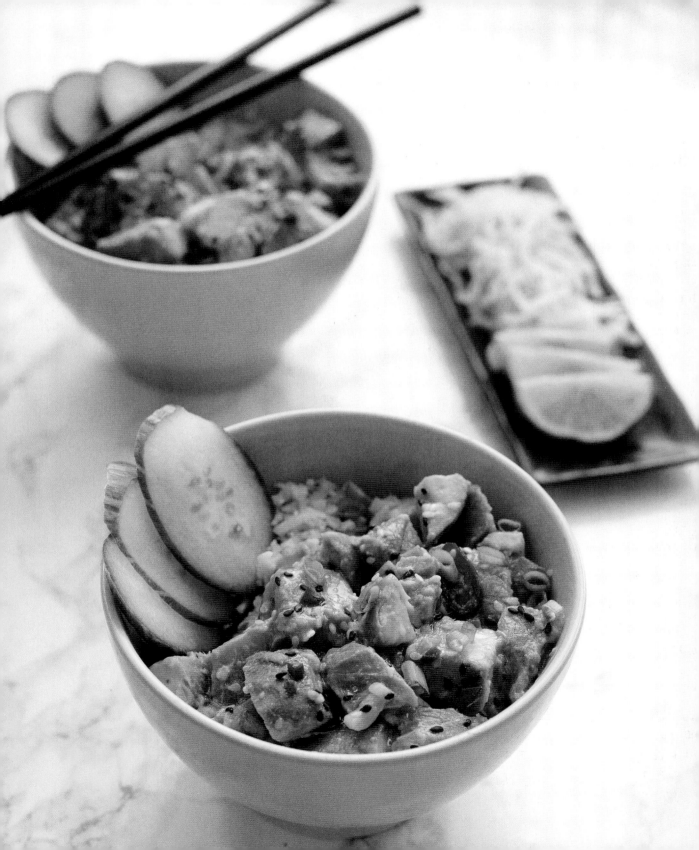

Tuna Poke Bowl

Here's my take on a popular Hawaiian summertime staple. The dish usually involves small pieces of raw fish marinated in soy sauce and served over rice. To make it suitable for keto and paleo diets, though, my recipe uses cauli-rice and coconut aminos in place of the traditional rice and soy sauce.

MAKES: 2 SERVINGS | HANDS-ON TIME: 20 MINUTES | OVERALL TIME: 25 MINUTES

MARINATED TUNA:

½ pound (225 g) sushi-grade tuna, skinless and boneless

2 tablespoons (30 ml/1 oz) each coconut aminos and extra-virgin olive oil

1 tablespoon (15 ml/0.5 oz) each toasted sesame oil and fresh lemon or lime juice

1 teaspoon rice vinegar or coconut vinegar

1 teaspoon Sriracha sauce

Salt

½ teaspoon grated fresh ginger, or ¼ teaspoon ground ginger

1 small chile pepper, sliced

2 medium (30 g/1.1 oz) spring onions, sliced

1 medium (150 g/5.3 oz) avocado, diced

1 tablespoon (9 g/0.3 oz) sesame seeds, divided

CAULI-RICE:

2 cups (240 g/8.5 oz) cauliflower rice (page 8)

1 tablespoon (15 g/0.5 oz) ghee or coconut oil

1 tablespoon (15 ml/0.5 oz) rice vinegar or coconut vinegar

¼ teaspoon salt, or to taste

TOPPING:

2 ounces (56 g) cucumber slices

To make the marinated tuna, cut the tuna into ½- to 1-inch (1 to 2 cm) pieces and place in a mixing bowl. In another bowl, mix the coconut aminos, olive oil, sesame oil, lemon juice, vinegar, Sriracha, and salt to taste. Add this mixture to the bowl with the tuna. Add the ginger, chile pepper, spring onions, and avocado. Add the sesame seeds, reserving 1 teaspoon for topping. Place in the fridge while you prepare the cauli-rice.

To make the cauli-rice, place the cauli-rice in a hot pan greased with the ghee. Cook over medium-high heat for 5 to 7 minutes. Stir to prevent burning. In a small bowl, mix the vinegar and salt. When the cauli-rice is done, remove from the heat, place in a bowl, and stir in the vinegar mixture.

To assemble, divide the cauli-rice between two bowls. Add the marinated tuna-and-avocado mixture. Top with the sliced cucumber and a sprinkle of the reserved sesame seeds.

NUTRITION FACTS PER SERVING

Total carbs: 17.6 g | Fiber: 8.6 g | Net carbs: 9 g | Protein: 32.8 g
Fat: 42 g | Energy: 565 kcal
Macronutrient ratio: Calories from carbs (7%), protein (24%), fat (69%)

Quick Salmon Patties

Fish cakes are healthy and easy to make, and they're versatile, too. You can use tuna, sardines, mackerel, or even white fish in place of the salmon, plus your favorite spices and herbs.

MAKES: 4 SERVINGS (12 PATTIES) | HANDS-ON TIME: 20 MINUTES | OVERALL TIME: 20 MINUTES

PATTIES:

1.1 pounds (500 g) canned salmon, drained

2 large pastured eggs

½ cup (50 g/1.8 oz) almond flour, or 2 tablespoons (16 g/0.6 oz) coconut flour

2 tablespoons (8 g/0.3 oz) chopped fresh parsley

1 tablespoon (4 g/0.1 oz) chopped fresh dill

1 tablespoon (15 ml/0.5 oz) fresh lemon juice

1 small (70 g/2.5 oz) white onion, finely chopped

1 clove garlic, crushed

1 teaspoon paprika

½ teaspoon each ground cumin and turmeric

Salt and pepper

2 tablespoons (30 g/1.1 oz) ghee, lard, or duck fat

AVOCADO & LIME DIP:

1 small (100 g/3.5 oz) avocado, peeled, seed removed

¼ cup (55 g/1.9 oz) Mayonnaise (page 20)

1 tablespoon (15 ml/0.5 oz) fresh lime juice

1 clove garlic, minced

1 tablespoon (4 g/0.1 oz) chopped fresh cilantro or parsley

Salt and pepper

Optional: leafy greens, extra-virgin olive oil, or avocado mayo

To make the patties, place all the ingredients except the ghee in a mixing bowl and combine. Scoop some of the salmon mixture into a ¼-cup measuring cup (about 58 g /2 oz) and press down with the back of a spoon to pack it tightly. Turn the measuring cup over onto a plate or a chopping board; repeat until you get 12 patties. Heat a large pan greased with the ghee over medium heat. Once hot, add as many patties as you can fit in a single layer. Cook on each side for 4 to 5 minutes and use a spatula to flip them over. (Do not force the patties out of the pan: If a patty doesn't release when you try to flip it, cook it for a few more seconds until it's crisp and ready to flip.) Set the cooked patties aside.

While the patties are cooking, prepare the avocado dip. Place all the ingredients in a blender. Process until smooth. Spoon into a serving bowl.

Serve the patties with the avocado dip and, optionally, a quick salad of leafy greens drizzled with extra-virgin olive oil or avocado mayo. To store, place the cooled patties and the avocado dip in separate airtight containers and refrigerate for up to 3 days.

NUTRITION FACTS PER SERVING (3 PATTIES + 2 TABLESPOONS DIP)

Total carbs: 8 g | Fiber: 3.7 g | Net carbs: 4.3 g | Protein: 39.9 g
Fat: 39.1 g | Energy: 532 kcal
Macronutrient ratio: Calories from carbs (3%), protein (30%), fat (67%)

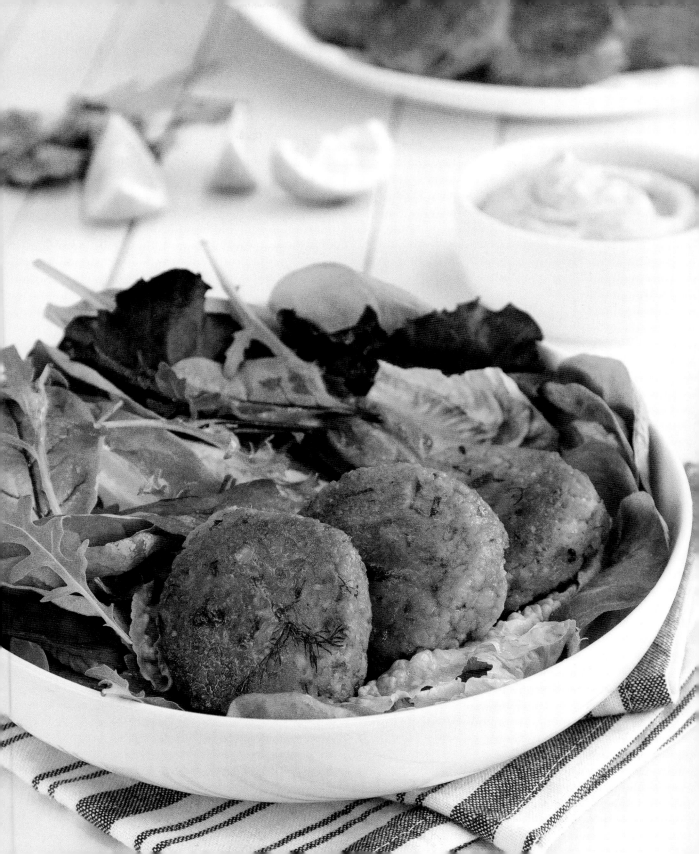

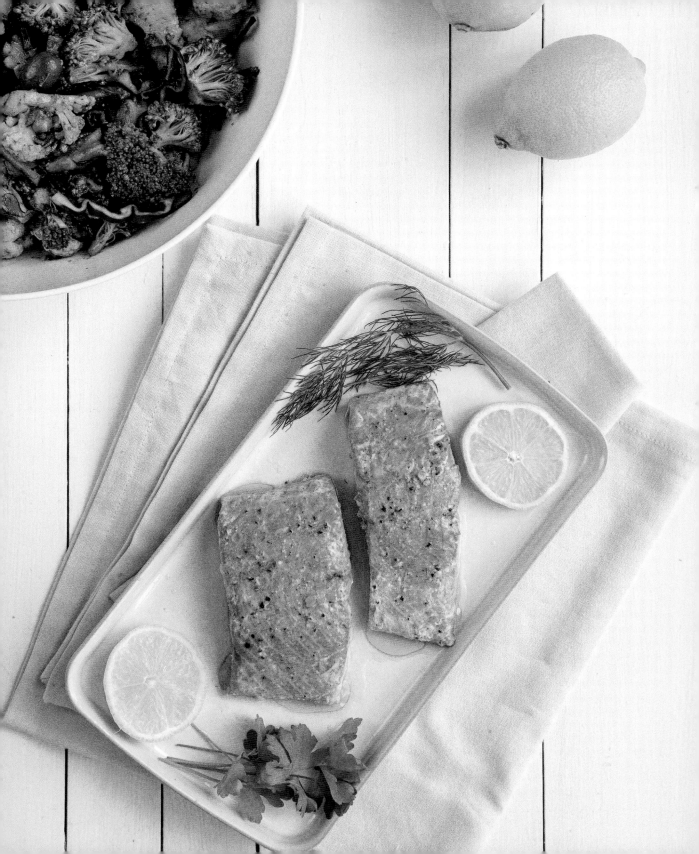

Poached Salmon with Broccoli Pesto Salad

Poaching is such an easy way to turn out perfectly cooked, juicy salmon every time. I like to serve mine with a warm, Italian-style broccoli salad.

MAKES: 4 SERVINGS | HANDS-ON TIME: 15 MINUTES | OVERALL TIME: 30 MINUTES

BROCCOLI PESTO SALAD:

½ medium (250 g/8.8 oz) cauliflower

1 small (250 g/8.8 oz) head broccoli

1 cup (70 g/2.5 oz) shredded red cabbage

2 tablespoons (17 g/0.6 oz) capers, drained

¼ cup (25 g/0.9 oz) pitted olives

¼ cup (60 g/2.1 oz) Avocado and Kale Pesto (page 19)

2 tablespoons (30 ml/1 oz) extra-virgin olive oil

Salt and pepper

POACHED SALMON:

½ cup (120 ml/4 oz) chicken stock or vegetable stock (page 13)

2 tablespoons (30 ml/1 oz) lemon juice

2 tablespoons (30 ml/1 oz) apple cider vinegar

1 small (70 g/2.5 oz) white onion, chopped

1 clove garlic, minced

1 small bunch fresh dill

1 small bunch parsley

4 medium (600 g/1.3 lb total) salmon fillets

Salt and pepper

2 tablespoons (30 ml/1 oz) extra-virgin olive oil

To make the salad, cut the cauliflower and broccoli into bite-size florets. Place the cauliflower in a steamer and cook for 2 minutes. Add the broccoli and cook for another 4 minutes, until the vegetables are crisp-tender. Remove from the heat and take off the lid. Place the cabbage into a mixing bowl. Add the steamed cauliflower and broccoli, capers, olives, pesto, and olive oil. Season with salt and pepper to taste, combine, and set aside.

To poach the salmon, heat the chicken stock, lemon juice, vinegar, onion, garlic, dill, and parsley in a large pan over medium heat. Season the salmon fillets with salt and pepper. When the liquid is simmering, add the salmon to it and cover with a lid. Reduce the heat to medium-low and cook for 7 to 10 minutes. Use a slotted spoon to transfer the cooked salmon to serving plates. Drizzle them with the olive oil, and serve with the prepared broccoli pesto salad. Discard the poaching liquid, or store in the fridge for up to 3 days and use for another batch.

NUTRITION FACTS PER SERVING

Total carbs: 10.9 g | Fiber: 4.3 g | Net carbs: 6.6 g | Protein: 36.9 g | Fat: 30.6 g | Energy: 462 kcal
Macronutrient ratio: Calories from carbs (6%), protein (33%), fat (61%)

Mediterranean Fish Bake

Packed with low-carb veggies, this one-tray meal is ideal for busy weeknights. Minimal cleanup required!

¼ cup (55 g/1.9 oz) ghee or duck fat, melted

2 cloves garlic, minced

1 small (200 g/7.1 oz) eggplant

2 medium (400 g/14.1 oz total) zucchini, sliced

1 medium (120 g/4.2 oz) bell pepper (red, orange, or yellow), sliced

1 bunch (150 g/5.3 oz) broccolini or regular broccoli florets

5.3 ounces (150 g) tomatoes, sliced

1 small (60 g/2.1 oz) red onion, sliced

¼ cup (10 g/0.4 oz) chopped fresh herbs (such as basil, oregano, thyme, parsley), divided

Salt and pepper

4 medium fillets (120 g/4.2 oz each) white fish, such as sea bass or sea bream

1 unwaxed lemon, sliced

2 tablespoons (30 ml/1 oz) extra-virgin olive oil

Preheat the oven to 400°F (200°C, or gas mark 6). Mix the ghee with the garlic. Roughly dice the eggplant into about 1-inch (2.5 cm) pieces. Place all the vegetables on a large baking tray. Sprinkle with the chopped herbs, reserving some for garnish. Season with salt and pepper, and drizzle with the prepared garlic ghee. Place in the oven and bake for about 15 minutes.

Add the fish fillets, seasoned with salt and pepper, skin-side up, and top with the lemon slices. Increase the temperature to 475°F (250°C, or gas mark 9). Place the baking tray back in the oven and, depending on the thickness of the fish, bake for 8 to 12 minutes, until the fillets are opaque. (You can use the broiler to crisp up the skin for the last few minutes of the cooking process, if you like.) Remove from the oven, and discard the lemon slices. Drizzle the fish with the olive oil, and sprinkle with the reserved herbs. To store, let it cool, transfer to an airtight container, and refrigerate for up to 3 days.

⌐ To make this recipe vegetarian, just replace the fish with the equivalent amount of Halloumi or feta cheese.

NUTRITION FACTS PER SERVING

Total carbs: 13.6 g | Fiber: 4.9 g | Net carbs: 8.7 g | Protein: 26.4 g | Fat: 32.5 g | Energy: 447 kcal
Macronutrient ratio: Calories from carbs (8%), protein (24%), fat (68%)

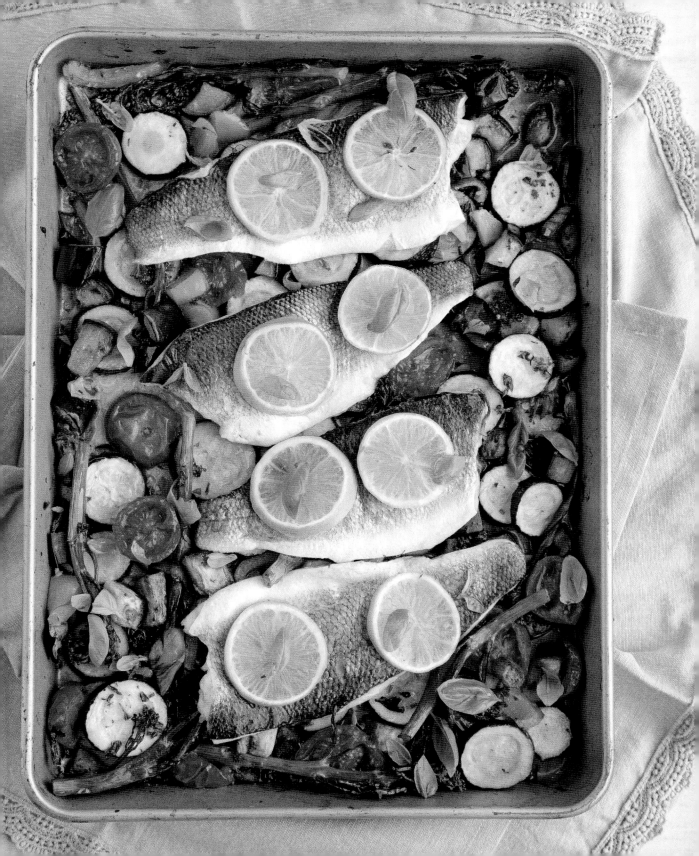

Seafood Risotto

There's no need to say good-bye to risotto just because you're eating low-carb. The secret here is cauli-rice. I always keep some prepped cauli-rice on hand in the fridge so that I can whip up this easy meal in a matter of minutes.

MAKES: 4 SERVINGS | HANDS-ON TIME: 15 MINUTES | OVERALL TIME: 15 MINUTES

2 tablespoons (30 g/1.1 oz) ghee or duck fat

3 ounces (85 g) Spanish chorizo or pepperoni, diced

1 small (70 g/2.5 oz) white or yellow onion, chopped

2 cloves garlic, minced

4 cups (480 g/16.9 oz) cauliflower rice (page 8)

4 cups (120 g/4.2 oz) chopped fresh spinach, or an equivalent amount of drained, cooked spinach

2 to 4 tablespoons (30 to 60 ml/ 1 to 2 oz) water or stock (page 13), if needed

7.1 ounces (200 g) cooked shrimp

7.1 ounces (200 g) cooked mussels, clams, squid, or a combination (frozen or canned)

1 tablespoon (15 ml/0.5 oz) fresh lemon juice

Salt and pepper

2 tablespoons (8 g/0.3 oz) chopped fresh parsley

¼ cup (60 ml/2 oz) extra-virgin olive oil

Optional: ½ cup (45 g/1.6 oz) grated Parmesan cheese

Heat a large pan greased with the ghee over medium-high heat. Add the chorizo, onion, and garlic. Cook until the chorizo is crisp and fragrant, 3 to 5 minutes. Add the cauliflower rice, reduce the heat to medium, and cook for 5 to 7 minutes. Add the water, if necessary.

Add the spinach and cook for 1 minute. Add the seafood of your choice and the lemon juice. Cook until heated through, 1 to 2 minutes. Season with salt and pepper to taste. Remove from the heat. To serve, top with the parsley, drizzle with the olive oil, and add the Parmesan (if using).

NUTRITION FACTS PER SERVING

Total carbs: 12.4 g | Fiber: 3.8 g | Net carbs: 8.6 g | Protein: 31.4 g | Fat: 39.6 g | Energy: 528 kcal
Macronutrient ratio: Calories from carbs (7%), protein (24%), fat (69%)

Healthy Deconstructed Hamburgers

I'd been cooking burgers the wrong way for years, until one day a friend of mine, a professional chef, shared the secret of his success with me. Simple preparation without overprocessing the meat is the best way to achieve juicy, evenly cooked burgers. But don't take my word for it: try them for yourself!

MAKES: 4 SERVINGS | HANDS-ON TIME: 15 MINUTES | OVERALL TIME: 20 MINUTES

BURGERS:

1.1 pounds (500 g) ground beef

Salt and pepper

1 tablespoon (15 g/0.5 oz) ghee or lard

Optional: 3 ounces (85 g) cheese of your choice (Cheddar, provolone, etc.)

BURGER SAUCE:

¼ cup (55 g/1.9 oz) Mayonnaise (page 20)

1 tablespoon (15 g/0.5 oz) sugar-free ketchup or tomato paste

1 teaspoon Dijon mustard

1 tablespoon (15 ml/0.5 oz) fresh lemon juice

1 tablespoon (20 g/0.7 oz) grated pickle

Salt and pepper

TOPPING:

1 large head (600 g/1.3 lb) iceberg lettuce

2 large (300 g/10.6 oz) tomatoes, sliced

8 small (200 g/7.1 oz) pickles

To make the burgers, gently divide the ground meat into 4 equal parts. Use your hands to shape each piece into a loose burger, about 4 inches (10 cm) in diameter. (Do not squeeze or pack the meat too tightly, or the burgers will lose their juiciness as they are cooked.) Season with salt and pepper on each side.

Heat a large pan greased with the ghee over high heat. Use a spatula to transfer the burgers to the hot pan. Cook for 3 minutes, then flip over with the spatula, and cook for an additional 2 to 3 minutes. If using cheese, place it on top of the burgers for the last minute of the cooking process. Set aside.

To make the burger sauce, mix the mayonnaise, ketchup, Dijon mustard, lemon juice, and pickle in a bowl. Season with salt and pepper to taste.

To assemble the burgers, tear off the lettuce leaves (allow about ¼ head per person), and place in serving bowls. Top with the burger and serve with tomatoes, pickles, and the prepared burger sauce.

Pimp your burger! Add any low-carb topping you like, such as sliced avocado, pickled onions, jalapeño peppers, Fresh Tomato Salsa (page 31), or Kimchi (page 24).

NUTRITION FACTS PER SERVING (1 BURGER + 2 TABLESPOONS BURGER SAUCE + VEGETABLES)

Total carbs: 9.4 g | Fiber: 3.4 g | Net carbs: 6 g | Protein: 24.1 g | Fat: 40.7 g | Energy: 497 kcal
Macronutrient ratio: Calories from carbs (5%), protein (20%), fat (75%)

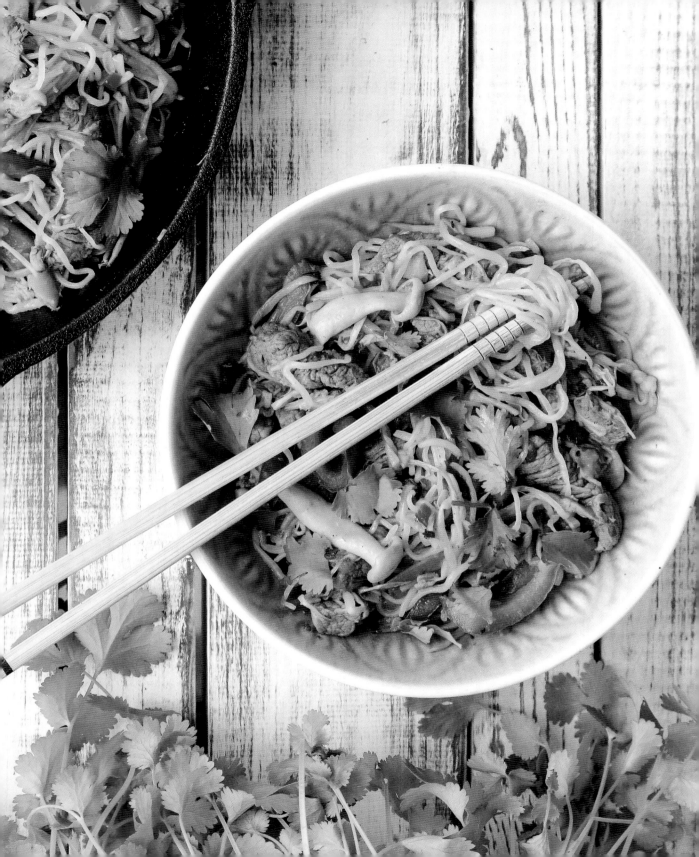

Beef Stir-Fry

You've got to try this fragrant, stick-to-your-ribs stir-fry. It features steak, low-carb vegetables, and keto-friendly shirataki noodles—and it takes barely half an hour to make.

MAKES: 4 SERVINGS | HANDS-ON TIME: 20 MINUTES | OVERALL TIME: 30 MINUTES

14.1 ounces (400 g) shirataki noodles, drained

2 medium (500 g/1.1 lb) sirloin steaks

¼ cup (55 g/1.9 oz) ghee, lard, or coconut oil, divided

Salt and pepper

2 cloves garlic, minced

1 small chile pepper, diced

1 tablespoon (6 g/0.2 oz) grated ginger

7.1 ounces (200 g) mixed Asian mushrooms (shiitake, oyster, and enoki) or brown mushrooms, sliced

2 medium (240 g/8.5 oz) green peppers, sliced

2 tablespoons (30 ml/1 oz) coconut aminos

2 tablespoons (30 ml/1 oz) fish sauce

2 cups (100 g/3.5 oz) bean sprouts

2 tablespoons (30 ml/1 oz) fresh lime or lemon juice

1 tablespoon (15 ml/0.5 oz) toasted sesame oil

2 medium (30 g/1.1 oz) spring onions, sliced

2 tablespoons (8 g/0.3 oz) chopped fresh cilantro or parsley

Wash the shirataki noodles thoroughly and boil for 2 to 3 minutes. Drain well. Place the noodles in a hot dry pan. Fry over medium-high heat for about 10 minutes. Using tongs, toss the noodles as they cook. (This step is important and ensures that the noodles won't be rubbery.) Place the fried noodles in a bowl and set aside.

Cut the steak into thin strips and place in a large, hot pan greased with 2 tablespoons (27.5 g/0.8 oz) of the ghee. Season with salt and pepper. Cook over medium-high heat, stirring occasionally until cooked through. Use a slotted spoon to transfer the steak to a plate.

Grease the pan in which you cooked the beef with the remaining 2 tablespoons (27.5 g/0.8 oz) ghee. Cook the garlic, chile pepper, and ginger over medium heat for 2 to 3 minutes, until fragrant. Add the mushrooms and cook for 5 minutes. Add the green peppers, coconut aminos, and fish sauce, and cook for 3 to 5 minutes more. Add the bean sprouts, cooked shirataki noodles, and cooked steak and cook until heated through, about 1 minute. Remove from the heat and add the lime juice, sesame oil, spring onions, and cilantro. Mix until well combined and serve immediately, or let cool and refrigerate for up to 3 days.

Shirataki noodles (also known as konjak noodles or konnyaku noodles) are popular in Asian cuisine. They're made from the konjak plant, which is ground and then shaped into noodles or even rice. Shirataki noodles are almost zero-calorie and zero-carb. They're 97 percent water, 3 percent fiber, and have traces of protein, fat, and calcium, and they can be used as part of a healthy low-carb diet.

NUTRITION FACTS PER SERVING
Total carbs: 11.8 g | Fiber: 4 g | Net carbs: 7.4 g | Protein: 28.9 g | Fat: 32.9 g | Energy: 449 kcal
Macronutrient ratio: Calories from carbs (7%), protein (26%), fat (67%)

Beef Fajitas

These Beef Fajitas require very little prep time
and make a speedy-yet-delicious dinner. Kids love them, too!

MAKES: 4 SERVINGS | HANDS-ON TIME: 20 MINUTES | OVERALL TIME: 20 MINUTES + MARINATING

MARINADE:

2 cloves garlic, minced

½ cup (120 ml/4 oz) extra-virgin olive oil

¼ cup (60 ml/2 oz) fresh lime juice

1 teaspoon cumin

1 teaspoon chili powder

½ teaspoon red pepper flakes

1 teaspoon salt, or to taste

¼ teaspoon ground black pepper

FAJITAS:

1 medium (110 g/3.9 oz) white or yellow onion, sliced

1 medium (120 g/4.2 oz) each red, orange, and yellow peppers (or 3 peppers of a single color), sliced

1 medium (120 g/4.2 oz) green bell pepper, sliced

1.3 pounds (600 g) flank steak (see note)

2 tablespoons (30 g/1.1 oz) ghee or lard, divided

2 small (200 g/7.1 oz) sliced avocados or Guacamole (page 122)

Optional: cheese (Cheddar, queso fresco, or feta), sour cream, Fresh Tomato Salsa (page 31), fresh cilantro, lime wedges

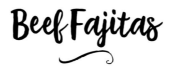

To make the marinade, mix all the ingredients in a bowl and set aside.

To make the fajitas, place the onion and peppers in another bowl, and the flank steak in a third bowl. Divide the marinade bet-ween the two bowls and toss to combine until the meat and vegetables are coated. Refrigerate for at least 1 hour or up to 24 hours.

When ready to cook, remove the steak from the marinade and pat dry. Set a large pan greased with 1 tablespoon (15 g/0.5 oz) of the ghee over high heat. Once hot, cook the steak for 2 to 3 minutes on each side, depending on the thickness, until medium-rare. Do not overcook the steak. Remove from the pan and keep warm.

Grease the same pan with the remaining 1 tablespoon (15 g/0.5 oz) ghee and place over high heat. Use a slotted spoon to add the vegetables to the pan. Cook for 3 to 5 minutes, stirring occasionally.

When ready to serve, slice the meat thinly against the grain. Serve with sliced avocados and the cooked onion and peppers. Optionally, serve with cheese, sour cream, salsa, cilantro, and lime wedges.

 You can use flank steak, skirt steak, or even sirloin steak for this recipe. While flank steak will take about 3 minutes per side to cook, skirt steak will take 2 to 3 minutes per side. If you're using thicker cuts like sirloin, follow the cooking instructions on page 105.

NUTRITION FACTS PER SERVING

Total carbs: 15 g | Fiber: 6.8 g | Net carbs: 8.2 g | Protein: 34.6 g | Fat: 33.1 g | Energy: 493 kcal
Macronutrient ratio: Calories from carbs (7%), protein (30%), fat (64%)

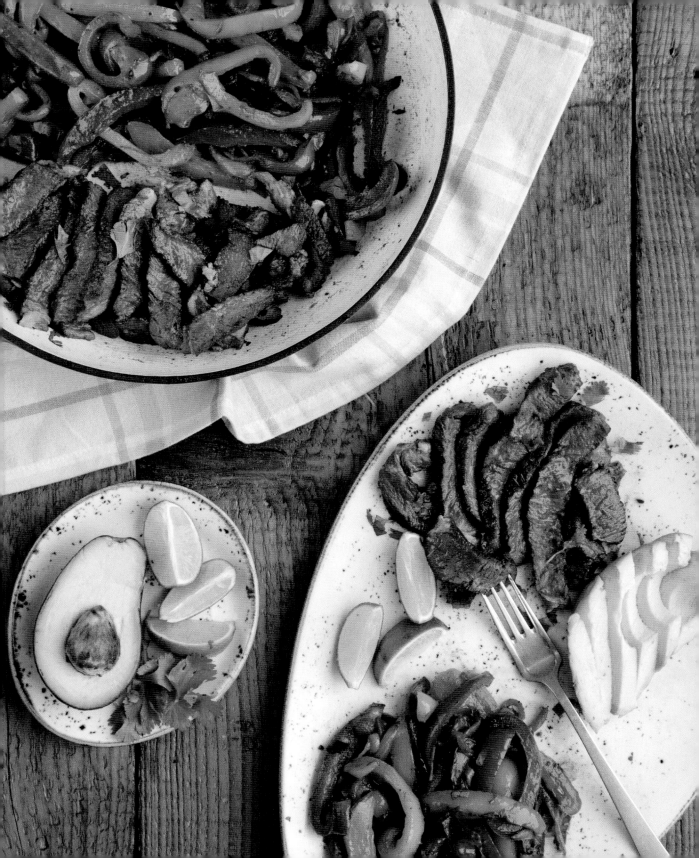

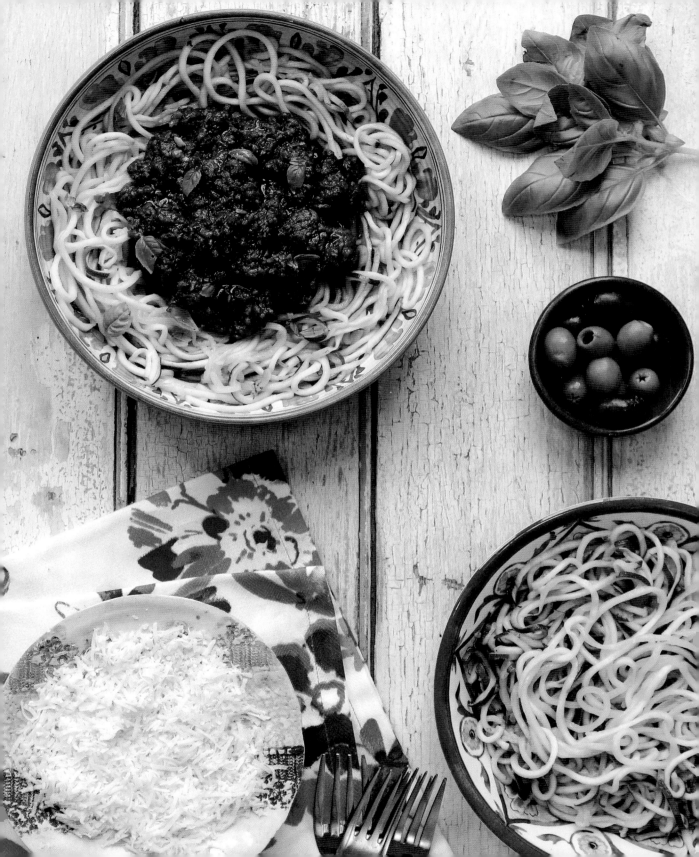

Beef Arrabiata Ragu

This is a low-carb take on penne arrabbiata, my favorite pasta dish. It's got just the right balance of flavors: a dash of spiciness from chile, plus lush sweetness from tomatoes. And, best of all, it takes just twenty minutes to make.

MAKES: 4 SERVINGS | HANDS-ON TIME: 20 MINUTES | OVERALL TIME: 20 MINUTES

4 medium (800 g/1.76 lbs) zucchini, spiralized (page 8)

½ teaspoon salt

2 tablespoons (30 g/1.1 oz) ghee or lard, divided

2 cloves garlic, minced

1.1 pounds (500 g) ground beef

1 cup (240 g/8.5 oz) unsweetened canned tomatoes

2 tablespoons (30 g/1.1 oz) unsweetened tomato paste

¼ cup (60 ml/2 oz) water or bone broth (page 13)

1 teaspoon red pepper flakes

2 teaspoons dried Italian herb mix

Salt and pepper

2 tablespoons (30 ml/1 oz) extra-virgin olive oil

Fresh basil

Optional: ½ cup (45 g/1.6 oz) grated Parmesan cheese

Sprinkle the spiralized zucchini "noodles" with salt and let them sit for 10 minutes. Use a paper towel to pat them dry. Set aside.

Prepare the ragu. Grease a large pan with 1 tablespoon (15 g/0.5 oz) of the ghee and place over medium-high heat. Add the garlic and cook for about 1 minute, until fragrant. Add the beef and cook until browned on all sides. Add the tomatoes, tomato paste, water, red pepper flakes, Italian herb mix, and salt and pepper to taste. Cook for 3 to 5 more minutes, until thickened, then remove from the heat.

Grease another pan with the remaining 1 tablespoon (15 g/0.5 oz) ghee. Cook the zucchini noodles for 2 to 5 minutes, tossing them in the pan while cooking. Serve the noodles topped with the prepared ragu, drizzled with the olive oil, and garnished with fresh basil. Optionally, sprinkle with grated Parmesan cheese.

NUTRITION FACTS PER SERVING

Total carbs: 10.9 g | Fiber: 3.3 g | Net carbs: 7.6 g | Protein: 24.8 g | Fat: 40.2 g | Energy: 500 kcal
Macronutrient ratio: Calories from carbs (6%), protein (20%), fat (74%)

Spinach Meatballs with Pesto Zoodles

These meatballs are so popular in my house that I usually make a couple of batches ahead of time and store them in the freezer so that I always have a quick dinner at the ready. Adding spinach to meatballs is a wonderfully sneaky way to get in extra vegetables at family meals, too!

MAKES: 4 SERVINGS | HANDS-ON TIME: 20 MINUTES | OVERALL TIME: 25 MINUTES

4 medium (800 g/1.76 lbs) zucchini

½ teaspoon salt

1.1 pounds (500 g) ground beef

3.5 ounces (100 g) cooked spinach, drained and chopped

1 large pastured egg

1 clove garlic, minced

2 tablespoons (8 g/0.3 oz) chopped fresh parsley

½ teaspoon salt

Ground black pepper

2 tablespoons (30 g/1.1 oz) ghee or lard, divided

½ cup (120 g/4.2 oz) Avocado and Kale Pesto (page 19)

Fresh basil

Optional: grated Parmesan cheese

Use a julienne peeler or a spiralizer to turn the zucchini into thin "noodles." Sprinkle the noodles with salt and let them sit for 10 minutes. Use a paper towel to pat them dry. Set aside.

Place the ground beef, spinach, egg, garlic, parsley, salt, and pepper to taste into a mixing bowl. Mix until well combined. Using your hands, create 20 meatballs (about 1 ounce/28 g each). Grease a large pan with 1 tablespoon (15 g/0.5 oz) of the ghee and place over medium heat. When hot, add the meatballs in a single layer. Cook for 2 minutes on each side, turning with a fork until browned on all sides and cooked through. Transfer the meatballs to a plate and keep warm.

Grease the same pan with the remaining 1 tablespoon (15 g/0.5 oz) ghee and cook the zucchini noodles for 2 to 5 minutes. Remove from the heat and mix in the pesto. Return the meatballs to the pan and add the fresh basil. Optionally, sprinkle with Parmesan cheese. Serve immediately. Store the meatballs in the fridge for up to 4 days, or freeze for up to 3 months.

NUTRITION FACTS PER SERVING (5 MEATBALLS + SAUCE + ZOODLES)

Total carbs: 9.9 g | Fiber: 4 g | Net carbs: 5.9 g | Protein: 27.6 g | Fat: 46 g | Energy: 558 kcal
Macronutrient ratio: Calories from carbs (4%), protein (20%), fat (76%)

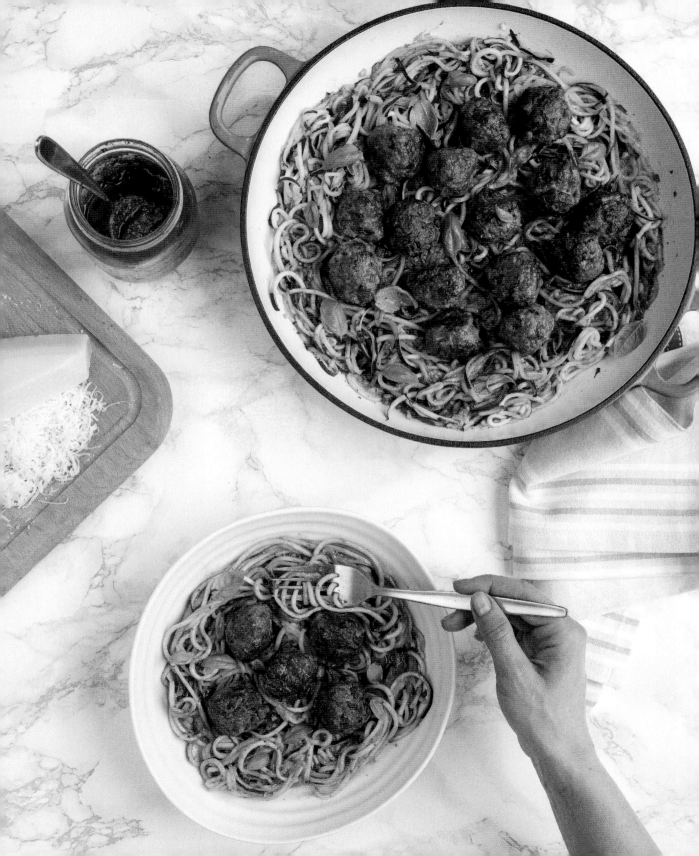

Pork Saltimbocca

Saltimbocca means "jumps in the mouth," and that's certainly true of this simple meal. A tasty variation of Italian chicken saltimbocca, it's served with lemon sauce and spinach—and it's ready in less than twenty minutes.

MAKES: 4 SERVINGS | HANDS-ON TIME: 20 MINUTES | OVERALL TIME: 20 MINUTES

SPINACH & MEDALLIONS:

1.3 pounds (600 g) fresh spinach or Swiss chard

1 pork tenderloin (500 g/1.1 lb)

Salt and pepper

8 fresh sage leaves

8 slices (120 g/4.2 oz) Parma ham

2 tablespoons (30 g/1.1 oz) ghee or lard

Optional: 3 ounces (85 g) provolone or mozzarella cheese, sliced

GRAVY:

½ cup (120 ml/4 oz) bone broth or chicken stock (page 13)

2 tablespoons (30 ml/1 oz) fresh lemon juice

⅓ cup (75 g/2.6 oz) butter or ghee

Salt and pepper

To make the spinach and medallions, bring a large pot of water to a boil and blanch the spinach for 30 to 60 seconds. Immediately plunge the spinach into a bowl filled with ice water. Drain well, pat dry, and set aside.

Cut the tenderloin into 8 medallions. Using a mallet, pound each medallion until about ¼-inch (½ cm) thick. (Alternatively, you can use boneless pork chops.) Season with salt and pepper. Place a fresh sage leaf in the middle of each piece and wrap each in a slice of Parma ham.

Heat a large pan greased with the ghee over medium-high heat. Add the medallions and cook for 6 to 8 minutes, flipping them over halfway through. Optionally, place half a slice of cheese on top of each medallion for the last 1 to 2 minutes of the cooking process. Transfer to a plate and keep warm.

To make the gravy, add the broth and lemon juice to the pan, stirring constantly. Add the butter, and season with salt and pepper to taste. Add the cooked spinach to the pan and stir to cover in the sauce. Alternatively, serve the sauce on the side, along with the medallions and spinach.

NUTRITION FACTS PER SERVING (2 MEDALLIONS + SPINACH)

Total carbs: 6.1 g | Fiber: 3.4 g | Net carbs: 2.7 g | Protein: 38.8 g | Fat: 30 g | Energy: 445 kcal
Macronutrient ratio: Calories from carbs (2%), protein (36%), fat (62%)

Pork Schnitzel with Zesty Slaw

Schnitzel was one of my favorite comfort foods when I was growing up in the Czech Republic, where it's served as part of the traditional Christmas feast. This recipe is pretty much as close as you can get to the real deal!

MAKES: 4 SERVINGS | HANDS-ON TIME: 25 MINUTES | OVERALL TIME: 25 MINUTES

SLAW:

10.6 ounces (300 g) green or white cabbage, shredded

7.1 ounces (200 g) red cabbage, shredded

⅓ cup (75 g/2.6 oz) Mayonnaise (page 20)

2 tablespoons (30 ml/1 oz) pickle juice or fresh lemon juice

2 medium (75 g/2.6 oz) pickles, grated

1 teaspoon Dijon mustard

½ teaspoon celery seed

1 tablespoon (4 g/0.1 oz) chopped fresh dill

1 tablespoon (4 g/0.1 oz) chopped fresh parsley

Salt and pepper

SCHNITZEL:

4 medium (600 g/1.3 lb total) boneless pork chops

Salt and pepper

1 large pastured egg

1 tablespoon (15 ml/0.5 oz) almond milk or water

½ cup (50 g/1.8 oz) almond flour

2.5 ounces (70 g) ground flaxseed

2 tablespoons (30 g/1.1 oz) ghee or lard

Chopped fresh parsley and lemon wedges

To make the slaw, place the green and red cabbage in a large bowl. In a small bowl, mix the mayonnaise, pickle juice, pickles, Dijon mustard, celery seed, dill, and parsley. Pour this mixture over the cabbage, and combine well. Season with salt and pepper to taste, mix again, and set aside.

To make the schnitzel, use a mallet to pound each pork chop to a thickness of ⅛- to ¼-inch (¼- to ½ cm). Season with salt and pepper on both sides. Crack the egg into a bowl, add the almond milk, and whisk with a fork. In another bowl, mix the almond flour and ground flaxseed. Dip each of the pork chops into the egg mixture, then dredge in the almond-and-flax mixture.

Heat a large pan greased with the ghee over medium heat. Once hot, cook the pork chops in a single layer for 3 to 4 minutes on each side, until golden brown. Serve warm with the prepared slaw, plus some fresh parsley and lemon wedges.

⌐ Make this recipe nut-free by substituting grated Parmesan cheese for the almond flour.

NUTRITION FACTS PER SERVING

Total carbs: 16.9 g | Fiber: 9.4 g | Net carbs: 7.5 g | Protein: 40.2 g
Fat: 48 g | Energy: 645 kcal
Macronutrient ratio: Calories from carbs (5%), protein (26%), fat (69%)

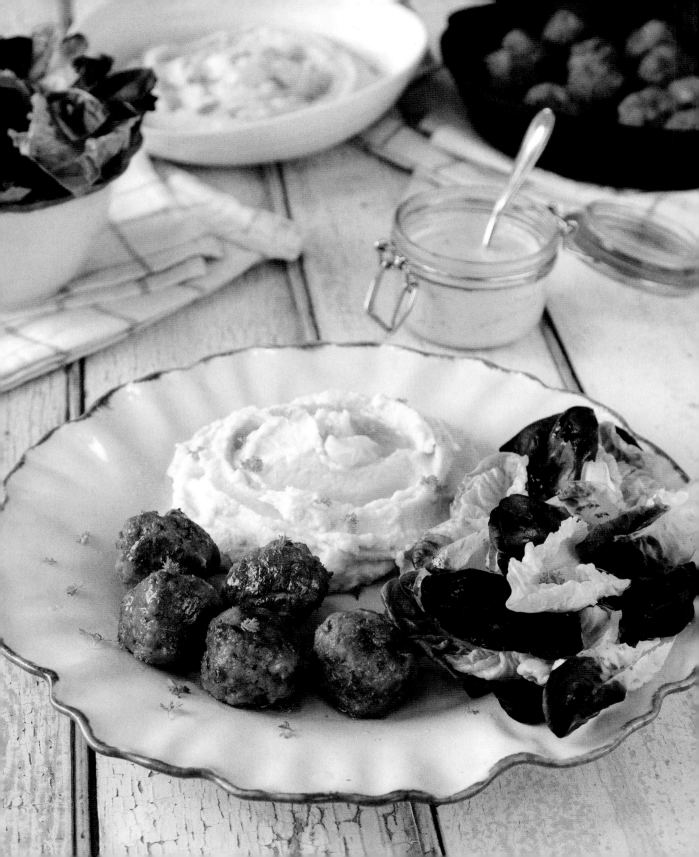

Czech Meatballs with Creamy Mash

Here's another traditional Czech recipe. This one is a tribute to my mom and dad, who passed their cooking skills—and their love of Czech cuisine—on to me. Most Czech meals are high in carbs, but I've transformed this one into a healthy, low-carb dinner that the whole family will love.

MAKES: 4 SERVINGS | HANDS-ON TIME: 30 MINUTES | OVERALL TIME: 30 MINUTES

MEATBALLS:

2 tablespoons (30 g/1.1 oz) ghee or lard

1 medium (110 g/3.9 oz) onion, chopped

2 cloves garlic, minced

1.1 pounds (500 g) ground pork

1 large pastured egg

½ cup (50 g/1.8 oz) almond flour

1 tablespoon (15 g/0.5 oz) Dijon mustard

2 teaspoons (4 g/0.1 oz) caraway seeds

1 tablespoon (1.7 g/0.1 oz) dried marjoram

2 teaspoons (5 g/0.16 oz) paprika

2 tablespoons (8 g/0.3 oz) chopped fresh parsley, plus more for garnish

½ teaspoon black pepper and salt

CAULIFLOWER MASH:

1 medium (600 g/1.3 lb) cauliflower

¼ cup (55 g/1.9 oz) butter or ghee, divided

Salt and pepper

OPTIONAL:

4 cups (120 g/4.2 oz) mixed salad greens

¼ cup (60 g/2.1 oz) tartar sauce (page 21)

To make the meatballs, heat a large pan greased with the ghee over medium-high heat. Add the onion and garlic, and cook until fragrant, about 3 minutes. Set aside. Place all the ingredients for the meatballs into a mixing bowl. Add the cooked onion and garlic. Mix until well combined. Set aside for a few minutes to allow the flavors to combine.

Meanwhile, prepare the cauliflower mash. Cut the cauliflower into medium-size florets and place in a steamer. Cook for about 10 minutes. Remove from the heat and place in a blender with 2 tablespoons (28 g/1 oz) of the butter, plus salt and pepper to taste. Process until smooth and set aside.

While the cauliflower is cooking, use your hands to shape the meat mixture into 20 medium-size meatballs. Grease the pan with the remaining 2 tablespoons (28 g/1 oz) butter. Once hot, add the meatballs in a single layer. Cook for 2 minutes per side, turning with a fork until browned on all sides and cooked through. Remove from the heat.

Serve, garnished with parsley, over the cauliflower mash. Optionally, add some leafy greens tossed with tartar sauce. To store, let the meatballs cool, then refrigerate them for up to 4 days, or freeze in a resealable plastic bag for up to 3 months.

NUTRITION FACTS PER SERVING (5 MEATBALLS + CAULI-MASH)

Total carbs: 14.8 g | Fiber: 5.9 g | Net carbs: 8.9 g | Protein: 29.3 g | Fat: 56.3 g | Energy: 674 kcal
Macronutrient ratio: Calories from carbs (5%), protein (18%), fat (77%)

Pork Stroganoff

Stroganoff is a traditional Russian stew that's often served with pasta—which, of course, is off-limits if you're following a ketogenic diet. The great news is that stroganoff also works well with low-carb vegetables such as asparagus, broccoli, green beans, or zucchini noodles.

MAKES: 4 SERVINGS | HANDS-ON TIME: 20 MINUTES | OVERALL TIME: 20 MINUTES

1.1 pounds (500 g) pork chops or tenderloin

Salt and pepper

2 tablespoons (30 g/1.1 oz) ghee or lard, divided

1 small (70 g/2.5 oz) white or yellow onion, chopped

2 cloves garlic, minced

3 cups (210 g/7.4 oz) sliced white mushrooms

1 cup (240 ml/8 oz) bone broth or chicken stock (page 13)

1 tablespoon (15 ml/0.5 oz) fresh lemon juice

1 tablespoon (15 g/0.5 oz) Dijon mustard

1 cup (240 ml/8 oz) heavy whipping cream or coconut milk

2 tablespoons (8 g/0.3 oz) chopped fresh parsley, plus more for garnish

1.1 pounds (500 g) asparagus

Slice the pork into thin strips. Season with salt and pepper. Heat a heavy-bottomed pan over high heat, and add 1 tablespoon (15 g/0.5 oz) of the ghee. Add the pork slices and quickly stir-fry them until browned. (Work in batches, if necessary. Do not overfill the pan.) Using a slotted spoon, transfer them to a plate and set aside.

Grease the pan with the remaining 1 tablespoon (15 g/0.5 oz) ghee. Add the onion and garlic. Cook until fragrant, about 3 minutes. Add the mushrooms, broth, lemon juice, Dijon mustard, and cream, and bring to a boil.

Cook for about 5 minutes, or until thickened. Remove from the heat, add the parsley, season with salt and pepper to taste, and set aside.

Bring a saucepan filled with salted water to a boil. Add the asparagus and cook for 1 to 2 minutes, until crisp-tender. Drain and serve with the pork stroganoff. Garnish with parsley. Serve immediately.

NUTRITION FACTS PER SERVING

Total carbs: 10.7 g | Fiber: 3.7 g | Net carbs: 7 g | Protein: 32.5 g | Fat: 42.8 g | Energy: 556 kcal
Macronutrient ratio: Calories from carbs (5%), protein (24%), fat (71%)

Pork & Radish Hash

With only six ingredients, this dish couldn't be easier to make, but it's surprisingly filling. It gets its Eastern European flavor from caraway and sauerkraut, which is super-healthy, by the way. (It supports the naturally occurring flora in your gut.)

MAKES: 4 SERVINGS | HANDS-ON TIME: 15 MINUTES | OVERALL TIME: 25 MINUTES

1.1 pounds (500 g) pork belly, sliced

½ cup (120 ml/4 oz) water

1.3 pounds (600 g) radishes, quartered

1 cup (142 g/5 oz) sauerkraut, drained

¼ teaspoon caraway seeds (omit if the sauerkraut already includes them)

Salt and pepper

2 tablespoons (8 g/0.3 oz) chopped fresh parsley or marjoram

NUTRITION FACTS PER SERVING

Total carbs: 6.8 g | Fiber: 3.5 g
Net carbs: 3.3 g | Protein: 13.1 g
Fat: 66.5 g | Energy: 679 kcal
Macronutrient ratio: Calories from carbs (2%), protein (8%), fat (90%)

Place the sliced pork belly in a large pan and add the water. Cook over medium-high heat until the water starts to boil. Reduce the heat to medium and cook until the water evaporates and the pork fat is rendered. Reduce the heat to low and cook until the meat is lightly browned and crispy, about 10 minutes. Remove the meat from the pan and let it cool slightly, then cut into pieces.

Add the radishes, sauerkraut, and caraway seeds to the pan. Season with salt and pepper, and cook for 5 to 10 minutes, until the radishes have softened slightly. Add the cooked pork belly back to the pan. Remove from the heat and add the parsley. Serve immediately, or let the hash cool and store it in an airtight container in the fridge for up to 4 days.

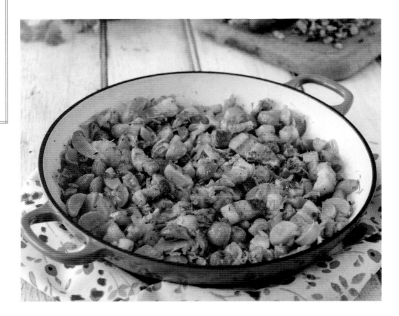

Tomato and Sausage Casserole

Another one-pot wonder! Here, I've turned the traditional Italian meal of sausages, peppers, and onions into a warming, tomato-based casserole that's especially cheering on wet, gloomy winter days.

MAKES: 4 SERVINGS | HANDS-ON TIME: 20 MINUTES | OVERALL TIME: 30 MINUTES

2 tablespoons (30 g/1.1 oz) ghee or lard, divided

1.1 pounds (500 g) gluten-free Italian sausages (4 to 8 links, depending on size)

1 small (70 g/2.5 oz) white or yellow onion, sliced

2 cloves garlic, minced

1 medium (120 g/4.2 oz) red pepper, sliced

1 medium (120 g/4.2 oz) green pepper, sliced

1½ cups (360 g/12.7 oz) unsweetened canned tomatoes

2 cups (140 g/5 oz) sliced white mushrooms

½ teaspoon red pepper flakes

2 teaspoons (2 g/0.07 oz) dried oregano

2 tablespoons (8 g/0.3 oz) chopped fresh parsley, divided

Salt and pepper

Preheat the broiler.

Heat a casserole dish greased with 1 tablespoon (15 g/0.5 oz) of the ghee over medium-high heat. Add the sausages and brown on all sides, about 5 minutes, turning with a fork. Transfer to a plate and set aside.

Grease the casserole dish with the remaining 1 tablespoon (15 g/0.5 oz) ghee. Add the onion and garlic. Cook for about 3 minutes, until fragrant. Add the red and green peppers and cook for another 3 minutes. Add the tomatoes, mushrooms, red pepper flakes, oregano, and parsley. (Reserve some parsley for garnish.) Bring to a boil and cook for 3 to 5 minutes. Place the sausages on top of the vegetables. Place the casserole under the broiler for 5 to 10 minutes, or until the sausages are browned and cooked through and the red sauce is bubbling. Set aside to cool for 5 minutes before serving. To store, let it cool and refrigerate in an airtight container for up to 4 days.

NUTRITION FACTS PER SERVING

Total carbs: 11.8 g | Fiber: 3.4 g | Net carbs: 8.4 g | Protein: 20.6 g | Fat: 47.2 g | Energy: 552 kcal
Macronutrient ratio: Calories from carbs (6%), protein (15%), fat (79%)

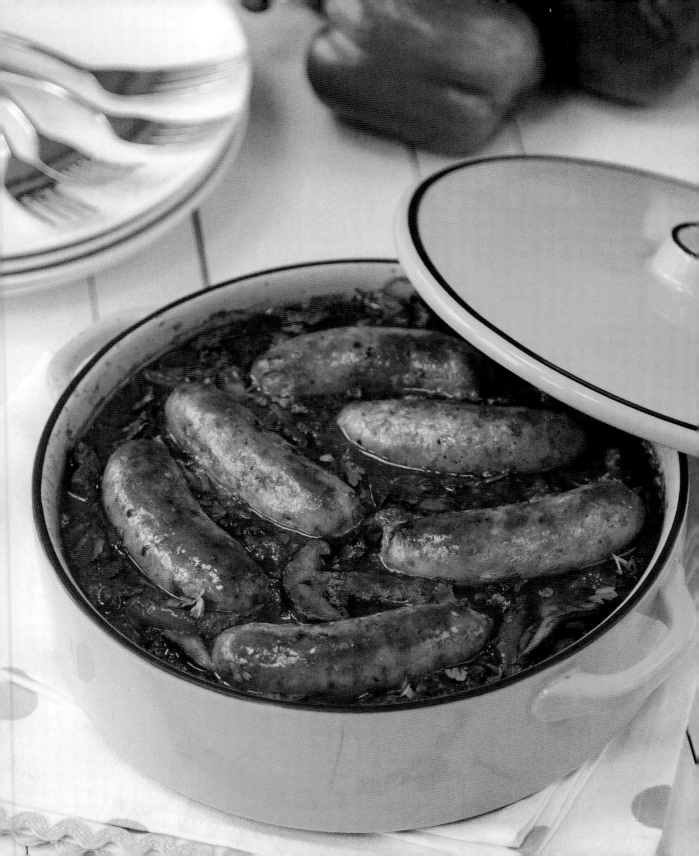

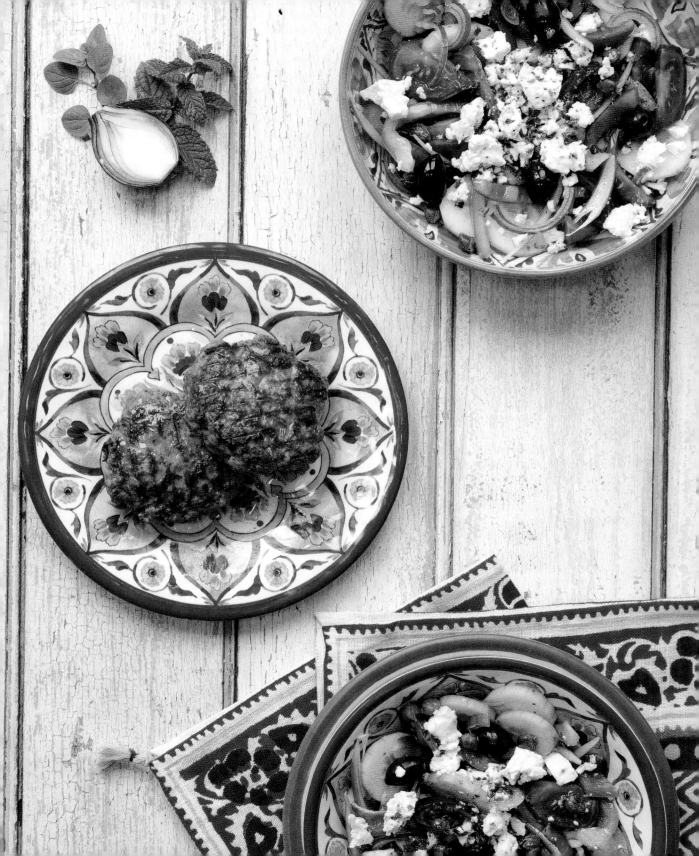

My Big Fat Greek Dinner

I make Mediterranean-inspired dishes almost every week—especially in the summer, when the warm weather seems to demand fresh, light flavors. Try these lamb burgers stuffed with feta cheese, plus a big bowl of Greek salad. It's one of our all-time favorite meals.

MAKES: 4 SERVINGS | HANDS-ON TIME: 30 MINUTES | OVERALL TIME: 30 MINUTES

FETA BURGERS:

1.1 pounds (500 g) ground lamb

1 small (60 g/2.1 oz) red onion, chopped

1 clove garlic, minced

1 tablespoon (4 g/0.1 oz) chopped fresh mint

1 teaspoon dried oregano

¼ teaspoon ground cumin

¼ teaspoon coriander

½ teaspoon salt

Black pepper

½ cup (75 g/2.6 oz) crumbled feta cheese

1 tablespoon (15 g/0.5 oz) ghee or lard

GREEK SALAD:

1 medium (250 g/8.8 oz) cucumber, sliced

10.6 ounces (300 g) tomatoes, sliced

1 medium (120 g/4.2 oz) green pepper, sliced

1 small (60 g/2.1 oz) red onion, sliced

¾ cup (112 g/4 oz) crumbled feta

16 olives (48 g/1.7 oz), pitted

Optional: 2 tablespoons (17 g/0.6 oz) capers, drained

1 teaspoon dried oregano

¼ cup (60 ml/2 oz) extra-virgin olive oil

To make the burgers, combine all the ingredients for the burgers, except the feta cheese and ghee, in a bowl. Using your hands, divide the mixture into 4 parts and flatten each until about ½ inch (1 cm) thick. Place one-fourth of the feta in the middle of each burger. Fold the meat over the cheese and press down on the sides to seal, shaping it into a patty. Cook on a hot pan greased with the ghee over medium-high heat for 5 to 6 minutes on each side. Set aside.

Meanwhile, prepare the salad. Place all the vegetables in a bowl and add the crumbled feta, olives, capers (if using), and oregano. Drizzle with the olive oil and serve with the feta burgers.

NUTRITION FACTS PER SERVING (1 BURGER + SALAD)

Total carbs: 11.5 g | Fiber: 3.2 g | Net carbs: 8.3 g | Protein: 30.2 g
Fat: 53 g | Energy: 635 kcal
Macronutrient ratio: Calories from carbs (5%), protein (19%), fat (76%)

Lamb Kebabs with Tabbouleh

Is there anything you can't do with cauli-rice? Here, I've turned it into a low-carb tabbouleh, which is the perfect complement to these Middle Eastern–style lamb kebabs.

MAKES: 4 SERVINGS | HANDS-ON TIME: 25 MINUTES | OVERALL TIME: 25 MINUTES

TABBOULEH:

1 tablespoon (15 g/0.5 oz) ghee or coconut oil

1 clove garlic, minced

4 cups (480 g/16.9 oz) cauliflower rice (page 8)

2 medium (200 g/7.1 oz) tomatoes, chopped

½ cup (30 g/1.1 oz) chopped fresh parsley, or to taste

¼ cup (15 g/0.5 oz) chopped fresh mint, or to taste

2 medium (30 g/1.1 oz) spring onions, sliced

¼ cup (60 ml/2 oz) fresh lemon juice

¼ cup (60 ml/2 oz) extra-virgin olive oil

Salt and pepper

KEBABS:

1.1 pounds (500 g) ground lamb

1 teaspoon onion powder

2 cloves garlic, minced

1 tablespoon (3 g/0.1 oz) dried oregano

1 teaspoon ground cumin

1 teaspoon paprika

½ teaspoon chili powder

¼ teaspoon ground allspice

¼ teaspoon black pepper

1 teaspoon salt

2 tablespoons (15 g/0.5 oz) ghee or coconut oil

To make the tabbouleh, heat a large pan greased with the ghee over medium-high heat. Add the garlic and cook until fragrant, 1 minute or less. Add the cauliflower rice and cook for about 5 minutes. Remove from the heat and let cool. Add the tomatoes, parsley, mint, spring onions, lemon juice, and olive oil. Stir and season with salt and pepper to taste.

To make the kebabs, place all the ingredients for the kebabs, except the ghee, in a bowl. Mix until well combined. Divide the meat mixture into 8 parts. Using your hands, form oval-shaped kebabs around each of 8 skewers. Heat a griddle pan greased with the ghee over medium-high heat. Place the skewers in the pan in a single layer and cook for 5 to 7 minutes, turning frequently, until browned on all sides and cooked through. Serve immediately, with the prepared tabbouleh. To store, let the kebabs and tabbouleh cool, and place into two separate containers. Store in the fridge for up to 4 days.

NUTRITION FACTS PER SERVING (2 KEBABS + TABBOULEH)

Total carbs: 13.5 g | Fiber: 4.9 g | Net carbs: 8.6 g | Protein: 25.3 g
Fat: 47.8 g | Energy: 569 kcal
Macronutrient ratio: Calories from carbs (6%), protein (18%), fat (76%)

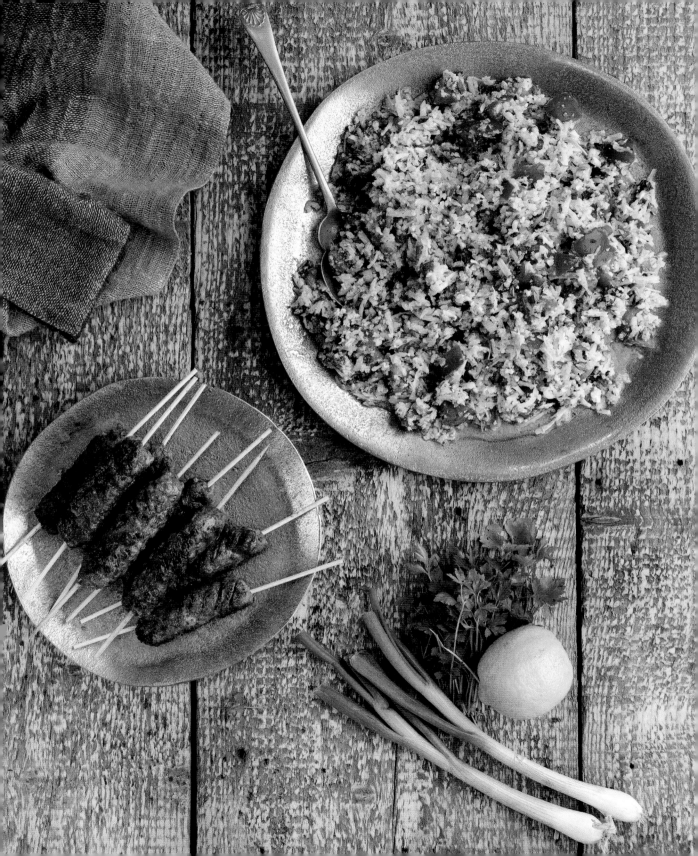

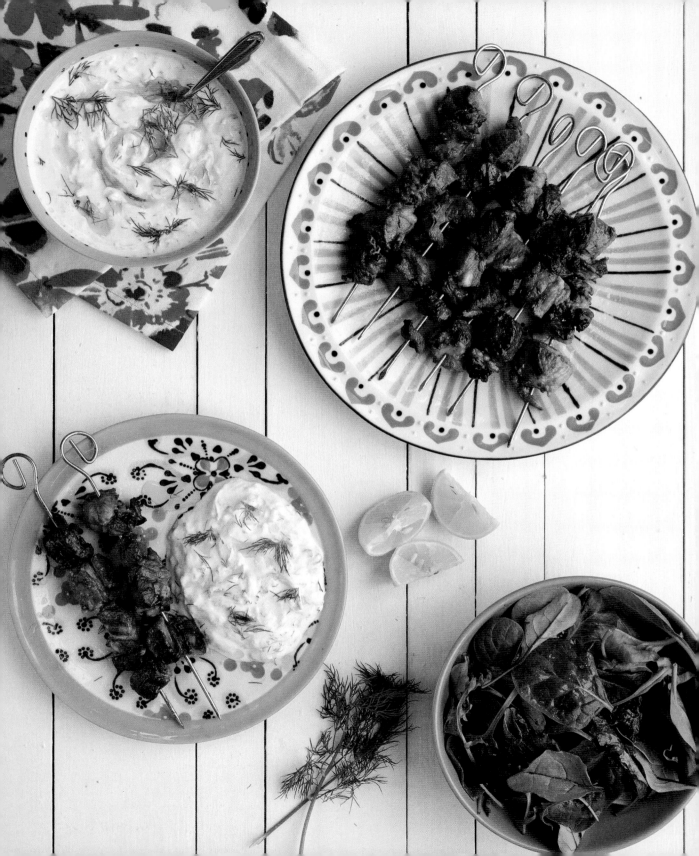

Lamb Souvlaki with Tzatziki

Souvlaki, or meat skewers, is one of the most popular dishes in Greece—not least because it requires minimum prep time. Tzatziki and Greek salad are both natural partners for it. (If you've never tried tzatziki, give it a shot. It's a savory herbed yogurt sauce, and it's delicious.)

MAKES: 4 SERVINGS (8 SKEWERS) | HANDS-ON TIME: 20 MINUTES | OVERALL TIME: 20 MINUTES + MARINATING

SOUVLAKI:

- 1.3 pounds (600 g) lamb leg or shoulder, cut into 2-inch (5 cm) chunks
- 1 small (70 g/2.5 oz) white or yellow onion, sliced
- 2 cloves garlic, minced
- ½ cup (30 g/1.1 oz) chopped mixed fresh herbs (like rosemary, mint, oregano, and thyme)
- ¼ cup (60 ml/2 oz) fresh lemon juice
- 1 cup (240 ml/8 oz) extra-virgin olive oil
- 1 teaspoon salt
- 1 tablespoon (15 g/0.5 oz) ghee or lard

TZATZIKI:

- 1 medium (200 g/7.1 oz) cucumber
- 2 cups (500 g/1.1 lb) full-fat yogurt
- 2 cloves garlic, minced
- 2 tablespoons (30 ml/1 oz) fresh lemon juice
- 1 teaspoon freshly grated lemon zest
- ¼ cup (60 ml/2 oz) extra-virgin olive oil
- 2 tablespoons (8 g/0.3 oz) chopped fresh dill
- Salt and pepper

To make the souvlaki, place the lamb chunks in a bowl. Add all the remaining ingredients except the ghee. Stir to coat the meat in the marinade. Cover with plastic wrap and refrigerate for at least 2 hours, or for up to 24 hours.

When you're ready to cook, thread the lamb chunks onto skewers, 4 per skewer. Reserve the marinade for another batch. (Store it in the fridge.) Heat a large griddle pan (or regular pan) greased with the ghee over medium-high heat. Once hot, add the skewers in a single layer and cook for 8 to 10 minutes, turning with a fork, until cooked through and browned on all sides.

Meanwhile, prepare the tzatziki. Grate the cucumber into a bowl. Add the yogurt, garlic, lemon juice, lemon zest, olive oil, and dill. Add salt and pepper to taste. Mix until combined. Serve immediately with the skewers, or store in an airtight container in the fridge for up to 3 days.

⌁ You can also make the skewers in the oven. Simply preheat the oven to 450°F (230°C, or gas mark 8) and bake for 15 to 20 minutes, turning halfway through.

NUTRITION FACTS PER SERVING (2 SKEWERS)

Total carbs: 6.9 g | Fiber: 0.3 g | Net carbs: 6.6 g | Protein: 39 g | Fat: 46 g | Energy: 601 kcal
Macronutrient ratio: Calories from carbs (4%), protein (26%), fat (69%)

CHAPTER 8:

Desserts and Drinks

Following a low-carb diet means sacrificing sugary treats. And, let's be honest, that's not always easy. Luckily, you don't need to avoid sweets altogether. There are plenty of healthy alternatives to reach for when cravings strike—like the high-fat, low-carb desserts in this chapter. In the pages that follow, you'll find keto-friendly versions of popular treats, including smoothies, ice cream, berry crumbles, lemon mousse, chia parfait, chewy cookies, fat bombs, brownies, and much more. Just remember that a dessert is still a dessert, even if it's low-carb. Try not to overdo it!

Tiramisu Mug Cake

This single-serving, low-carb tiramisu—which means "pick me up" in Italian—is healthier than the original. It's faster, too. Ten minutes is all you need.

MAKES: 1 SERVING | HANDS-ON TIME: 10 MINUTES | OVERALL TIME: 10 MINUTES

MUG CAKE:

2 heaping tablespoons (16 g/0.6 oz) almond flour

1 heaping tablespoon (12 g/0.4 oz) coconut flour

⅛ teaspoon baking soda

1 tablespoon (10 g/0.4 oz) powdered erythritol or Swerve, or 3 to 5 drops liquid stevia extract

1 large pastured egg

1 tablespoon (15 ml/0.5 oz) coconut oil or butter, melted

COFFEE LIQUID:

⅓ cup (80 ml/2.7 oz) prepared coffee

1 tablespoon (10 g/0.4 oz) powdered erythritol or Swerve, or 3 to 5 drops liquid stevia extract

¼ teaspoon unsweetened rum extract

TOPPING:

1 heaping tablespoon (30 g/1.1 oz) mascarpone cheese or creamed coconut milk (page 10)

2 heaping tablespoons (20 g/0.7 oz) unsweetened whipped cream, or 1 tablespoon (15 ml/0.5 oz) unwhipped cream

Optional: 3 to 5 drops liquid stevia extract

½ teaspoon unsweetened cacao powder

1 small square (5 g/0.2 oz) dark chocolate (85% cacao or more), grated

To make the cake, place the almond flour, coconut flour, baking soda, and erythritol into a mug or a ramekin. Combine well. Add the egg and coconut oil, and mix well with a fork. Microwave on high for 60 to 90 seconds.

Remove the mug from the microwave and let it cool for a couple of minutes. Remove the cake from the mug and halve widthwise.

To make the coffee liquid, mix the coffee and erythritol; add the rum extract. Use a spoon to soak both halves of the cake in the coffee liquid.

To make the topping, mix the mascarpone with the whipped cream and stevia (if using). Spread half of the topping on the cut cake. Place the other half of the cake on top and spread with the remaining topping. Dust with the cacao powder and top with the grated dark chocolate.

⌁ To make the recipe nut-free, use 1 level tablespoon (8 g/0.3 oz) of coconut flour instead of 2 tablespoons (16g/0.6 oz) of almond flour.

⌁ If you don't have a microwave, you can make 4 to 8 servings at once in the oven. Preheat the oven to 350°F (175°C, or gas mark 4). Make each serving in an individual ovenproof ramekin. Place the ramekins on a baking tray and transfer to the oven. Cook for 12 to 15 minutes, or until lightly browned and set. Then, follow the instructions for the coffee liquid and topping.

NUTRITION FACTS PER SERVING

Total carbs: 10.8 g | Fiber: 4.4 g | Net carbs: 6.4 g
Protein: 14.8 g | Fat: 49.1 g | Energy: 538 kcal
Macronutrient ratio: Calories from carbs (5%), protein (11%), fat (84%)

Fat-Fueled Smoothie Two Ways

Keto smoothies like this Fat-Fueled Smoothie are my go-to breakfast meals. They're ideal for busy mornings!

MAKES: 1 SERVING | HANDS-ON TIME: 5 MINUTES | OVERALL TIME: 5 MINUTES

BASE INGREDIENTS

½ large (100 g/3.5 oz) avocado

¼ cup (60 ml/2 oz) coconut milk

¾ to 1 cup (180 to 240 ml/6.1 to 8 oz) water, plus a few ice cubes

Optional: liquid stevia extract, powdered erythritol, or Swerve

FOR A CHOCOLATE SMOOTHIE:

1 tablespoon (16 g/0.6 oz) coconut butter or almond butter

1 tablespoon (5 g/0.2 oz) unsweetened cocoa powder, or raw cacao

½ teaspoon ground cinnamon

FOR A BERRY SMOOTHIE:

½ cup (75 g/2.6 oz) fresh or frozen berries (raspberries, blackberries, or strawberries)

¼ teaspoon vanilla powder or ½ teaspoon unsweetened vanilla extract

Place all the base and flavor-specific ingredients in a blender, including the sweetner (if using). Pulse until smooth. Serve immediately.

↻ VARIATIONS:

Get creative and add any of these ingredients to my basic Fat-Fueled Smoothie.

- 1 tablespoon (15 ml/0.5 oz) MCT oil gives you an extra energy boost.
- 2 tablespoons (15 g/0.5 oz) of collagen powder or 1 scoop quality protein powder helps you stay full for longer.
- 1 cup (30 g/1.1 oz) of fresh spinach is a great way to sneak more greens into your diet!
- 1 tablespoon (8 g/0.3 oz) chia seeds adds fiber and produces a thicker texture.
- 1 to 2 tablespoons (16 to 32 g/0.6 to 1.1 oz) of any nut or seed butters, or coconut butter, contributes a creamy texture, plus fiber, protein, and healthy fats.
- 1 to 2 teaspoons maca powder boosts energy levels, strengthens your immune system, and increases stamina and libido. It's high in phytochemicals. Maca is also a powerful adaptogen; that is, it helps our bodies to adapt to—and avoid damage from—environmental factors such as stress, poor diet, and toxins.

NUTRITION FACTS PER SERVING (CHOCOLATE SMOOTHIE)

Total carbs: 17.7 g | Fiber: 11.6 g | Net carbs: 6.1 g | Protein: 5.2 g | Fat: 36.3 g | Energy: 377 kcal
Macronutrient ratio: Calories from carbs (6%), protein (6%), fat (88%)

NUTRITION FACTS PER SERVING (BERRY SMOOTHIE)

Total carbs: 16.4 g | Fiber: 8.8 g | Net carbs: 7.6 g | Protein: 3.9 g | Fat: 27 g | Energy: 301 kcal
Macronutrient ratio: Calories from carbs (10%), protein (5%), fat (85%)

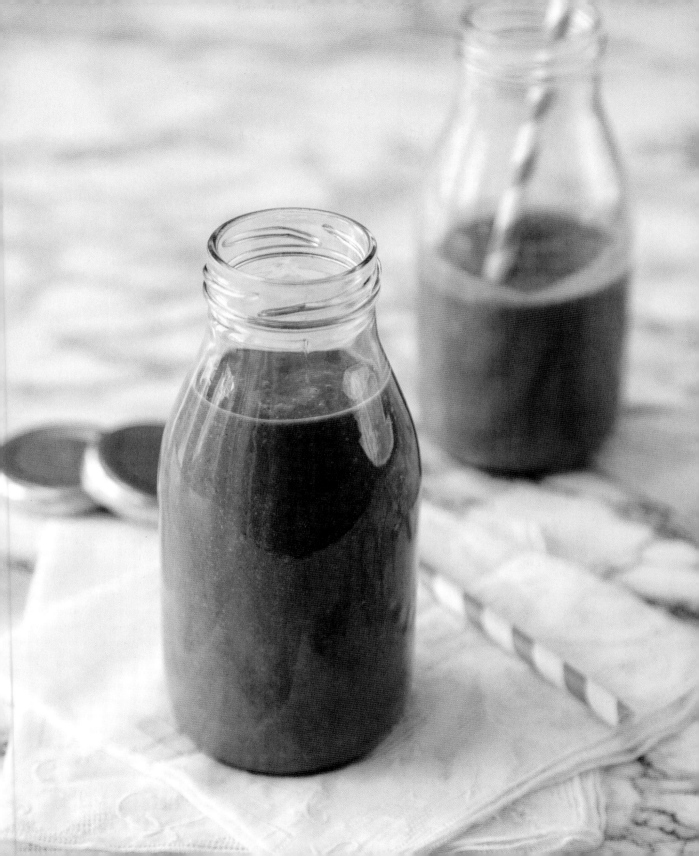

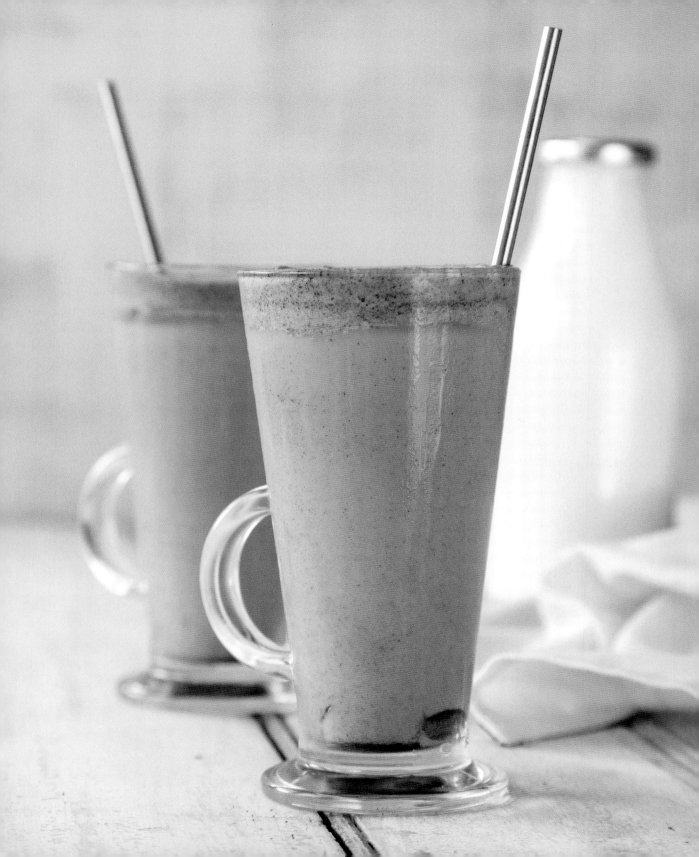

Iced Vanilla Latte

Use either chilled tea or coffee plus coconut milk to make this clean, refreshing, iced vanilla latte. Add a tablespoon of collagen, if you like. It'll help you stay full for longer.

⅔ cup (160 ml/5.4 oz) prepared coffee or black tea, cooled

¼ cup (60 ml/2 oz) coconut milk, or 2 tablespoons (30 ml/1 oz) heavy whipping cream

¼ teaspoon vanilla powder or 1 teaspoon unsweetened vanilla extract

1 tablespoon (15 ml/0.5 oz) MCT oil or macadamia oil

A few ice cubes

Optional: 1 tablespoon (10 g/ 0.4 oz) erythritol or Swerve, or 3 to 5 drops liquid stevia extract

Optional: 2 tablespoons (15 g/0.5 oz) collagen powder

Combine all the ingredients in a blender, including the sweetener and collagen powder (if using). Pulse until smooth. Serve in a glass over more ice cubes.

NUTRITION FACTS PER SERVING

Total carbs: 1.7 g | Fiber: 0 g | Net carbs: 1.7 g | Protein: 1.3 g | Fat: 25.7 g | Energy: 233 kcal
Macronutrient ratio: Calories from carbs (3%), protein (2%), fat (95%)

Blender Berry Ice Cream

All you need to whip up this satisfying, low-carb ice cream is five minutes and a few basic low-carb ingredients. To make it even more filling, add a scoop of quality protein powder or collagen.

MAKES: 2 SERVINGS | HANDS-ON TIME: 5 MINUTES | OVERALL TIME: 5 MINUTES

1 cup (120 g/4.2 oz) mascarpone cheese or creamed coconut milk (page 10)

1 cup (150 g/5.3 oz) mixed frozen berries

1 teaspoon unsweetened vanilla extract or ¼ teaspoon vanilla powder

2 tablespoons (30 ml/1 oz) MCT oil

Optional: 3 to 5 drops liquid stevia extract

Place all the ingredients into a blender, plus a dash of water if the mixture seems too thick. Pulse until smooth. Serve immediately—there's no need to freeze it first before eating! Or freeze in an airtight container for up to 3 months. To serve after freezing, leave the frozen ice cream at room temperature for 10 to 15 minutes to soften. (I like to use single-serving containers; they make serving simple, and they're great for portion control.)

～ You can use coconut or macadamia oil instead of MCT oil. If you're using coconut oil, be sure to blend the ice cream especially well. (Unlike MCT oil, coconut oil solidifies at low temperatures.)

NUTRITION FACTS PER SERVING

Total carbs: 7.2 g | Fiber: 2 g | Net carbs: 5.2 g | Protein: 4.2 g | Fat: 35 g | Energy: 359 kcal
Macronutrient ratio: Calories from carbs (6%), protein (5%), fat (89%)

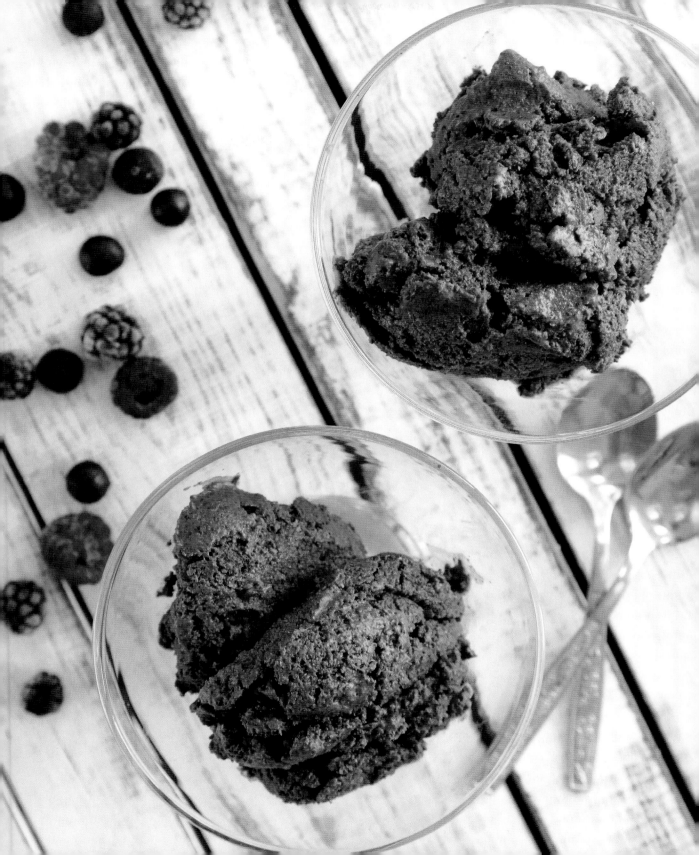

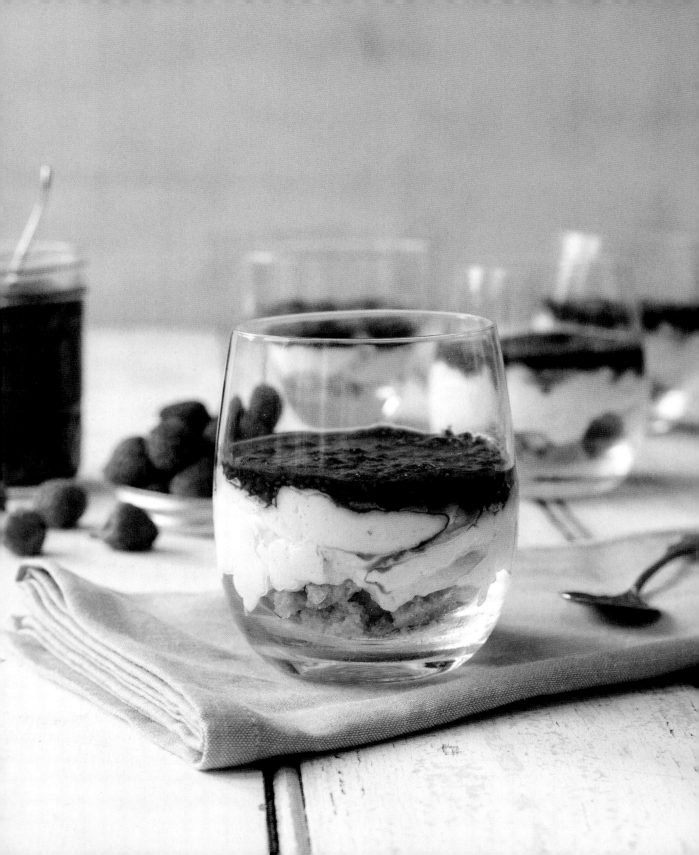

Raspberry Cheesecake in a Jar

Stored and served in individual jars or glasses, these no-bake cheesecakes are a quick and easy treat. Featuring a homemade, low-carb cookie "crust" and a layer of Raspberry Chia Jam, they're one of the most popular keto treats in my house!

MAKES: 4 SERVINGS | HANDS-ON TIME: 15 MINUTES | OVERALL TIME: 30 MINUTES

CRUST:

½ cup (50 g/1.8 oz) almond flour

1 tablespoon (15 g/0.5 oz) butter, ghee, or coconut oil

¼ teaspoon ground cinnamon

1 tablespoon (10 g/0.4 oz) erythritol or Swerve, or 3 to 5 drops liquid stevia extract

CHEESECAKE LAYER:

1 cup (240 g/8.5 oz) full-fat cream cheese or creamed coconut milk (page 10)

1 cup (240 ml/8 oz) heavy whipping cream or liquid coconut milk

2 tablespoons (30 ml/1 oz) fresh lemon juice

½ teaspoon vanilla powder or 1 to 2 teaspoons unsweetened vanilla extract

¼ cup (40 g/1.4 oz) powdered erythritol or Swerve, or 15 to 20 drops liquid stevia extract

TOPPING:

½ cup (160 g/5.6 oz) Raspberry Chia Jam (page 29) or equivalent amount of crushed raspberries

To make the crust, preheat the oven to 350°F (175°C, or gas mark 4). Mix all the ingredients for the crust in a bowl. Place the dough on a baking sheet lined with parchment paper. Using your hands, press down and flatten the dough to create a large cookie, about ⅛ inch (25 mm) thick. Transfer to the oven and bake for 8 to 10 minutes, or until golden brown. Remove from the oven and set aside to cool for 10 minutes.

Meanwhile, prepare the cheesecake layer. Combine the cream cheese, cream, lemon juice, vanilla, and erythritol in a bowl. Beat with an electric mixer or whisk.

When ready to assemble, crumble the cookie into smaller pieces and divide among 4 jars. Top each with the prepared cheesecake layer and Raspberry Chia Jam. Serve, or store in the fridge, covered with plastic wrap, for up to 3 days.

To make this recipe nut-free, try a combination of shredded unsweetened coconut and ground sunflower seeds instead of almond flour.

NUTRITION FACTS PER SERVING

Total carbs: 12 g | Fiber: 4.3 g | Net carbs: 7.7 g | Protein: 8.9 g | Fat: 49.9 g | Energy: 500 kcal
Macronutrient ratio: Calories from carbs (6%), protein (7%), fat (87%)

Blackberry Lemon Mousse

Studded with juicy blackberries, this light and
airy lemon mousse is the ultimate post-barbecue dessert.

MAKES: 5 SERVINGS | HANDS-ON TIME: 25 MINUTES | OVERALL TIME: 30 MINUTES

4 large pastured eggs

½ cup (120 ml/4 oz) fresh lemon juice

1 tablespoon (6 g/0.2 oz) finely grated lemon zest (1 to 2 lemons)

⅓ cup (50 g/1.8 oz) powdered erythritol or Swerve

Optional: liquid stevia extract

1 cup (240 ml/8 oz) heavy whipping cream or creamed coconut milk (page 10)

1½ cups (180 g/6.4 oz) blackberries

In a bowl, whisk 2 whole eggs and 2 egg yolks (reserve the whites for later). Add the lemon juice, lemon zest, and powdered erythritol, and combine. Set the bowl over a saucepan of simmering water, making sure that the water doesn't touch the bowl. Cook over medium-high heat, stirring constantly, until thickened, about 10 minutes. Then, take off the heat and set aside for 5 minutes. Pour the lemon curd into a bowl set over a larger bowl filled with ice water. Stir for about 5 minutes, or until chilled. Taste and add a few drops of stevia for more sweetness, if you like.

Place the egg whites in another bowl and beat with an electric mixer until stiff peaks form. Gently fold in the cooled lemon curd. In a separate bowl, whip the cream until firm, then fold it gently into the lemon curd mixture. This is the lemon mousse. Place a few blackberries into 5 serving bowls, divide the mousse among them, and top with the remaining blackberries. Serve, or cover the bowls with plastic wrap and refrigerate for up to 3 days.

NUTRITION FACTS PER SERVING

Total carbs: 7.4 g | Fiber: 2.1 g | Net carbs: 5.3 g | Protein: 6.5 g | Fat: 22.3 g | Energy: 256 kcal
Macronutrient ratio: Calories from carbs (8%), protein (11%), fat (81%)

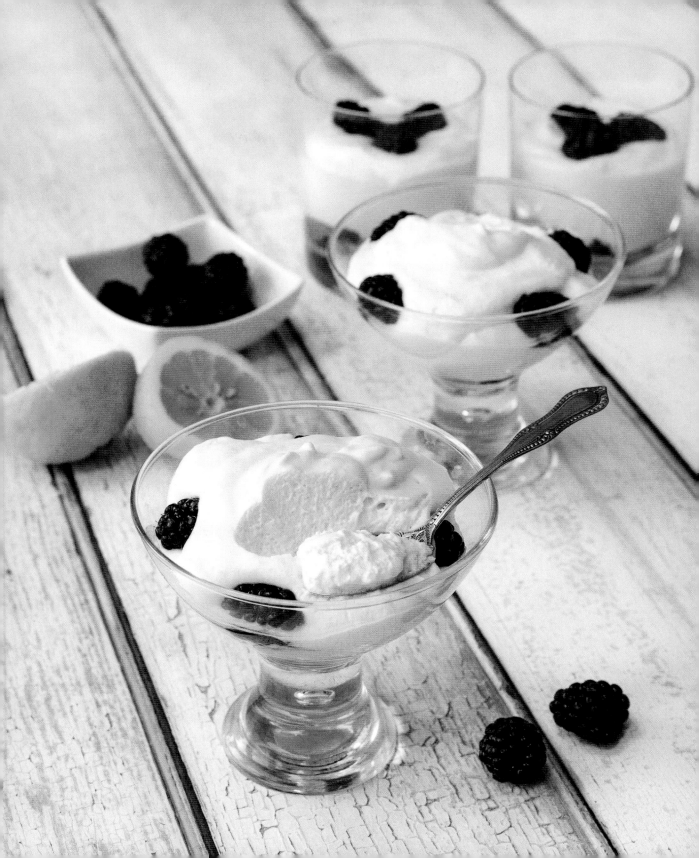

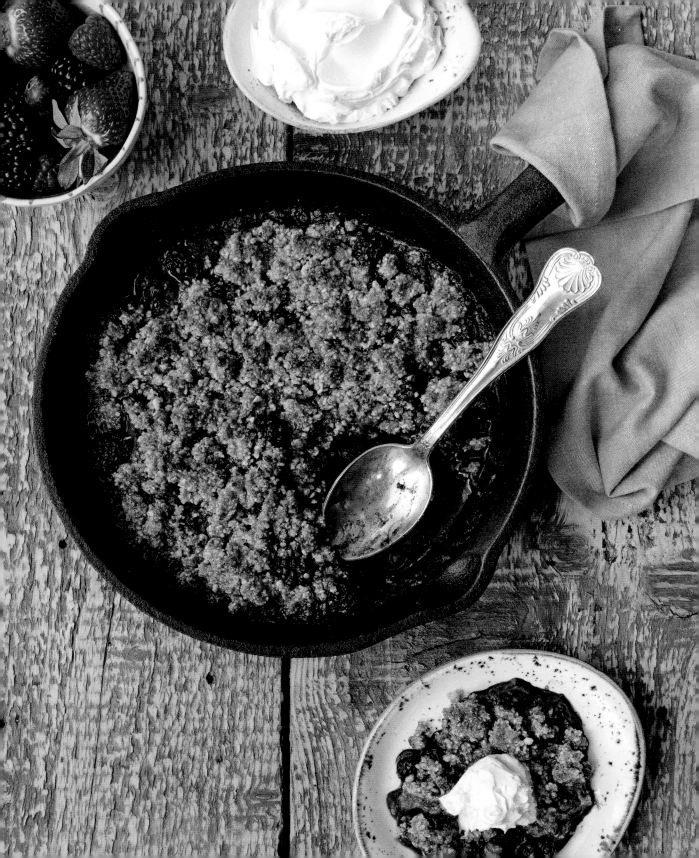

Skillet Berry Crumble

This simple crumble is truly a one-dish wonder,
and it's a great way to use up your stock of late-summer berries.

MAKES: 6 SERVINGS | HANDS-ON TIME: 10 MINUTES | OVERALL TIME: 25 MINUTES

BERRY BASE:

1 tablespoon (15 g/0.5 oz) ghee or coconut oil

2 cups (300 g/10.6 oz) mixed berries (raspberries, blackberries, strawberries, and/or blueberries), fresh or frozen

Optional: 5 to 10 drops liquid stevia extract

CRUMBLE:

1 cup (140 g/5 oz) almonds

½ cup (55 g/1.9 oz) pecans

2 tablespoons (30 g/1 oz) butter or coconut oil

1 teaspoon cinnamon or vanilla powder

¼ teaspoon salt

Optional: 2 tablespoons (20 g/0.7 oz) erythritol or Swerve, or 5 to 10 drops liquid stevia extract

Preheat the oven to 400°F (200°C, or gas mark 6).

To make the berry base, heat a medium-size skillet greased with the ghee over medium-high heat. Add the berries and cook for 3 to 5 minutes, until softened. Taste and add stevia if desired. Set aside.

Place the almonds and pecans (preferably soaked and dehydrated [page 11]) into a food processor. Add the butter, cinnamon, salt, and erythritol (if using). Pulse for a few seconds until the mixture is chopped as roughly or as finely as you like.

Sprinkle the nut mixture on top of the berries and broil for about 10 minutes, until lightly browned and crisp on top. Transfer to a cooling rack and let cool for 5 minutes. Serve warm or cold with a dollop of mascarpone cheese, sour cream, full-fat yogurt, or creamed coconut milk (page 10) flavored with vanilla extract.

⌒ You can make this crumble with any kind of nuts (macadamia, walnuts, or hazelnuts), seeds (sunflower, hemp, or pumpkin), or even shredded unsweetened coconut.

NUTRITION FACTS PER SERVING

Total carbs: 10.8 g | Fiber: 5.3 g | Net carbs: 5.5 g | Protein: 6.4 g | Fat: 24.8 g | Energy: 275 kcal
Macronutrient ratio: Calories from carbs (8%), protein (10%), fat (82%)

Strawberry and Rhubarb Fool

This one's a definite crowd-pleaser and with good reason.
The luscious strawberries and sweet whipped cream in this fruit-laden fool
bring back happy childhood memories of long, warm summer nights.

MAKES: 4 SERVINGS | HANDS-ON TIME: 10 MINUTES | OVERALL TIME: 20 MINUTES

FRUIT LAYER:

1 cup (150 g/5.3 oz) strawberries, fresh or frozen, halved

1¼ cups (150 g/5.3 oz) sliced fresh rhubarb

2 tablespoons (20 g/0.7 oz) erythritol or Swerve, or 5 to 10 drops liquid stevia extract

1 teaspoon cinnamon

CREAM LAYER:

1¼ cups (300 ml/10.1 oz) heavy whipping cream or creamed coconut milk (page 10)

¼ teaspoon vanilla powder or 1 teaspoon unsweetened vanilla extract

Optional: 2 tablespoons (20 g/0.7 oz) powdered erythritol or Swerve, or 5 to 10 drops liquid stevia extract

To make the fruit layer, place the strawberries, rhubarb, erythritol, and cinnamon in a medium saucepan. Cook over medium heat for 5 to 10 minutes, or until softened, crushing with a fork to speed the process. When the fruit is soft, set aside to cool for 10 minutes. (To speed cooling, you can set the saucepan over a bowl filled with ice water.)

To make the cream layer, in a bowl, whip the cream with the vanilla and erythritol (if using) until firm. Place alternating layers of fruit mixture and whipped cream into each of 4 serving glasses. Serve immediately, or cover the glasses with plastic wrap and refrigerate for up to 3 days.

NUTRITION FACTS PER SERVING

Total carbs: 7.4 g | Fiber: 1.8 g | Net carbs: 5.6 g | Protein: 2 g | Fat: 28.7 g | Energy: 297 kcal
Macronutrient ratio: Calories from carbs (8%), protein (3%), fat (89%)

Quick Skillet Brownie

This no-fuss skillet brownie is nut-free—and it's a guilt-free treat for us die-hard chocoholics, too!

MAKES: 8 SERVINGS | HANDS-ON TIME: 5 MINUTES | OVERALL TIME: 20 MINUTES

⅓ cup (75 g/2.6 oz) butter or coconut oil, melted, divided

2 large pastured eggs

¼ cup (60 ml/2 oz) prepared coffee, or almond milk

½ cup (43 g/1.5 oz) unsweetened cocoa powder or raw cacao

2 tablespoons (16 g/0.6 oz) ground chia seeds

⅓ cup (50 g/1.8 oz) powdered erythritol or Swerve

1 teaspoon cinnamon or vanilla powder

⅛ teaspoon salt

2 teaspoons (9 g/0.3 oz) gluten-free baking powder

Optional: 10 to 20 drops liquid stevia extract

Preheat the oven to 350°F (175°C, or gas mark 4). In a bowl, mix the melted butter (reserve 1 teaspoon for greasing), eggs, and coffee. Add the cocoa powder, chia seeds, erythritol, cinnamon, salt, and baking powder. If you prefer your brownie on the sweet side, add a few drops of stevia.

Pour the dough into an 8-inch (20 cm) skillet greased with ghee or an 8 x 8-inch (20 x 20 cm) parchment-lined pan. Transfer to the oven and bake for 12 to 15 minutes for fudgy brownies, or up to 18 minutes for cake-like ones. (Do not overbake: the brownie will continue to cook when left in the hot pan.) Test for doneness by inserting a toothpick into the center of the brownie. (The center should be just set.) Remove from the oven and set aside to cool. Cut into 8 slices and serve. Store at room temperature for up to 4 days, or freeze in an airtight container for up to 6 months.

⌒ It's easy to make your own gluten-free baking powder. For every teaspoon of baking powder, use a mixture of ¼ teaspoon of baking soda plus ½ teaspoon of cream of tartar or apple cider vinegar.

NUTRITION FACTS PER SERVING

Total carbs: 4.9 g | Fiber: 2.7 g | Net carbs: 2.2 g | Protein: 3.1 g | Fat: 10.2 g | Energy: 111 kcal
Macronutrient ratio: Calories from carbs (8%), protein (11%), fat (81%)

Chewy Pumpkin and Chocolate Chip Cookies

Rich, spicy, and addictive, these chewy cookies are a
perfect match for mid-morning coffee or tea.

MAKES: 10 SERVINGS | HANDS-ON TIME: 10 MINUTES | OVERALL TIME: 25 MINUTES

1 cup (250 g/8.8 oz) almond butter or sunflower seed butter

1 large pastured egg

⅓ cup (65 g/2.3 oz) unsweetened pumpkin purée

1 tablespoon (8 g/0.3 oz) pumpkin pie spice mix

2 tablespoons (20 g/0.7 oz) erythritol or Swerve

Optional: 5 to 10 drops liquid stevia extract

¼ teaspoon salt

½ cup (90 g/3.2 oz) dark chocolate chips or roughly chopped chocolate (85% cacao or more)

Preheat the oven to 350°F (175°C, or gas mark 4). Place all the ingredients except the chocolate chips into a food processor. Pulse until smooth. Scoop the cookie dough into a bowl and add the chocolate chips. Mix well with a wooden spoon.

Line a baking sheet with parchment paper. Using a spoon or a cookie scoop, create 10 mounds of dough. Place them on the parchment-lined tray, and flatten each with a fork or spoon. Bake for 13 to 15 minutes, until lightly golden and cooked through. Transfer to a wire rack to cool. (The cookies will crisp up slightly as they cool.) Store in an airtight container for up to a week, or freeze for up to 3 months.

NUTRITION FACTS PER SERVING (1 COOKIE)

Total carbs: 8.4 g | Fiber: 4.4 g | Net carbs: 4 g | Protein: 6.4 g | Fat: 17.1 g | Energy: 224 kcal
Macronutrient ratio: Calories from carbs (8%), protein (13%), fat (79%)

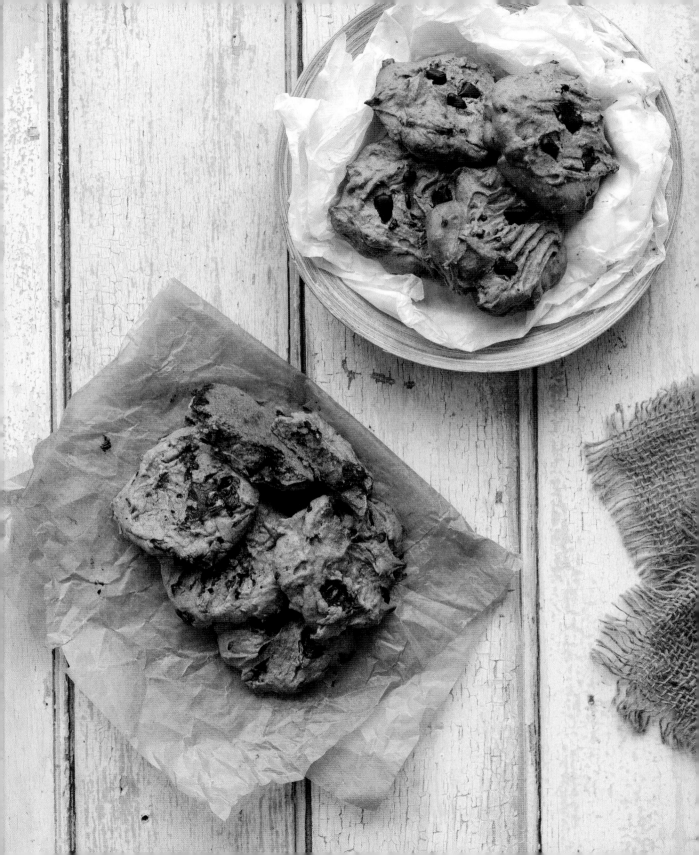

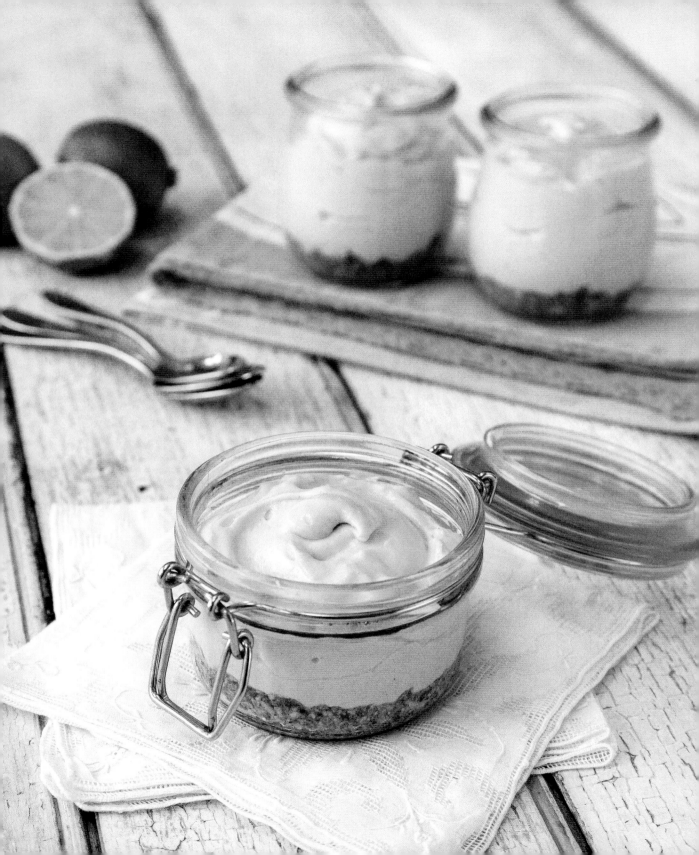

Key Lime Pie in a Jar

There's a secret ingredient in this recipe: avocado! And that's not as weird as it sounds. With its neutral taste and creamy texture, avocado is a blank canvas for strongly flavored ingredients such as lime juice or chocolate. It's also a great way to sneak heart-healthy, monounsaturated fats into desserts.

MAKES: 4 SERVINGS | HANDS-ON TIME: 15 MINUTES | OVERALL TIME: 15 MINUTES

CRUST:

⅓ cup (25 g/0.9 oz) unsweetened shredded coconut

⅓ cup (50 g/1.8 oz) almonds or sunflower seeds

1 tablespoon (15 g/0.5 oz) butter or coconut oil

¼ teaspoon salt

½ teaspoon vanilla powder, or 1 to 2 teaspoons unsweetened vanilla extract

1 tablespoon (10 g/0.4 oz) erythritol or Swerve, or 3 to 5 drops liquid stevia extract

LIME LAYER:

1 large (200 g/7.1 oz) avocado

1 cup (240 g/8.5 oz) mascarpone cheese or creamed coconut milk (page 10)

⅓ cup (80 ml/2.7 oz) fresh lime juice

1 teaspoon finely grated lime zest

¼ cup (40 g/1.4 oz) powdered erythritol or Swerve, or 15 to 20 drops liquid stevia extract

To make the crust, place the coconut in a hot dry skillet and fry for 1 to 2 minutes, stirring frequently, until fragrant. Add the coconut, almonds, butter, salt, vanilla, and erythritol (if using) to a food processor. Process until the mixture is chopped as roughly or as finely as you like, then divide it among 4 jars.

To make the lime layer, halve the avocado and remove the seed. Scoop the avocado flesh into a blender with the mascarpone cheese, lime juice, lime zest, and erythritol. Process until smooth. Place an equal amount of the mixture into each jar on top of the crusts. Serve immediately, or cover the jars with plastic wrap and store in the fridge for up to 3 days.

NUTRITION FACTS PER SERVING

Total carbs: 11.8 g | Fiber: 6 g | Net carbs: 5.8 g | Protein: 8.4 g | Fat: 38.4 g | Energy: 418 kcal
Macronutrient ratio: Calories from carbs (6%), protein (8%), fat (86%)

Candied Spiced Cocoa Pecans

You know a dessert is a winner when your guests devour it in mere minutes. I made a batch of these Candied Spiced Cocoa Pecans for some friends during the holiday season, and the pecans were gone before I even turned around!

MAKES: 8 SERVINGS (400 G/14 OZ) | HANDS-ON TIME: 5 MINUTES | OVERALL TIME: 30 MINUTES

2 large egg whites

¼ teaspoon salt

¼ cup (40 g/1.4 oz) powdered erythritol or Swerve

2 teaspoons (2 g) pumpkin pie spice mix or cinnamon

¼ cup (20 g/0.7 oz) unsweetened cacao powder or raw cacao

3½ cups (350 g/12.3 oz) pecans, preferably activated (page 10)

Preheat the oven to 300°F (150°C, or gas mark 2). Whisk the egg whites in a bowl until frothy. Gradually add the salt, erythritol, pumpkin pie spice, and cocoa powder. Add the pecans, and stir until they're completely coated in the mixture.

Spread the nuts in a single layer on a large baking tray lined with parchment paper and transfer to the oven. Bake for 15 to 20 minutes, until crispy. Remove from the oven and use a spatula to break the nut mixture into pieces while still warm. Let cool, then store in an airtight container for up to a month.

🥄 Use your leftover egg yolks to make Mayonnaise (page 20) or Quick Béarnaise Sauce (page 23).

NUTRITION FACTS PER SERVING (½ CUP/50 G/1.8 OZ)

Total carbs: 8.3 g | Fiber: 5.4 g | Net carbs: 2.9 g | Protein: 5.4 g | Fat: 31.9 g | Energy: 314 kcal
Macronutrient ratio: Calories from carbs (4%), protein (7%), fat (89%)

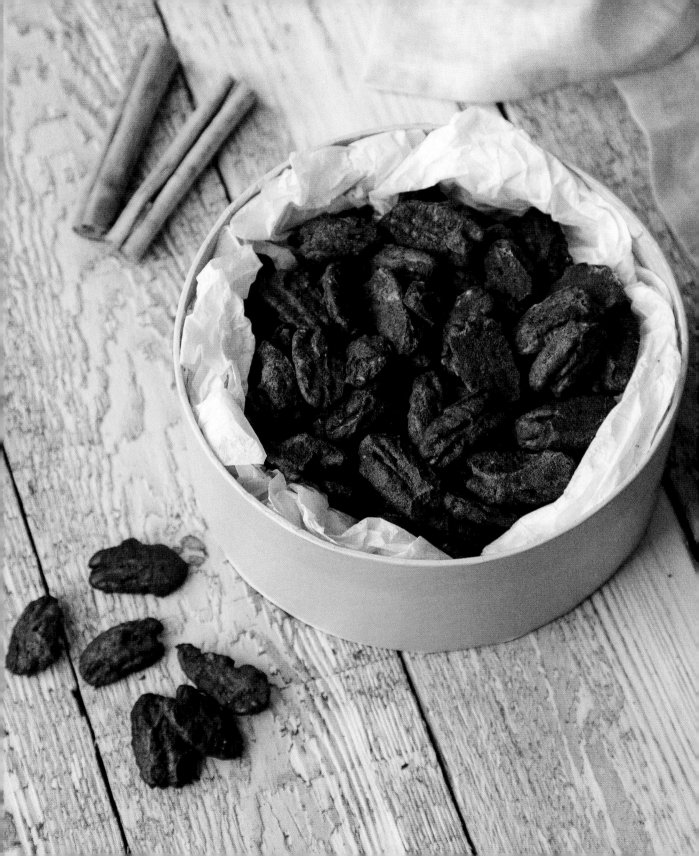

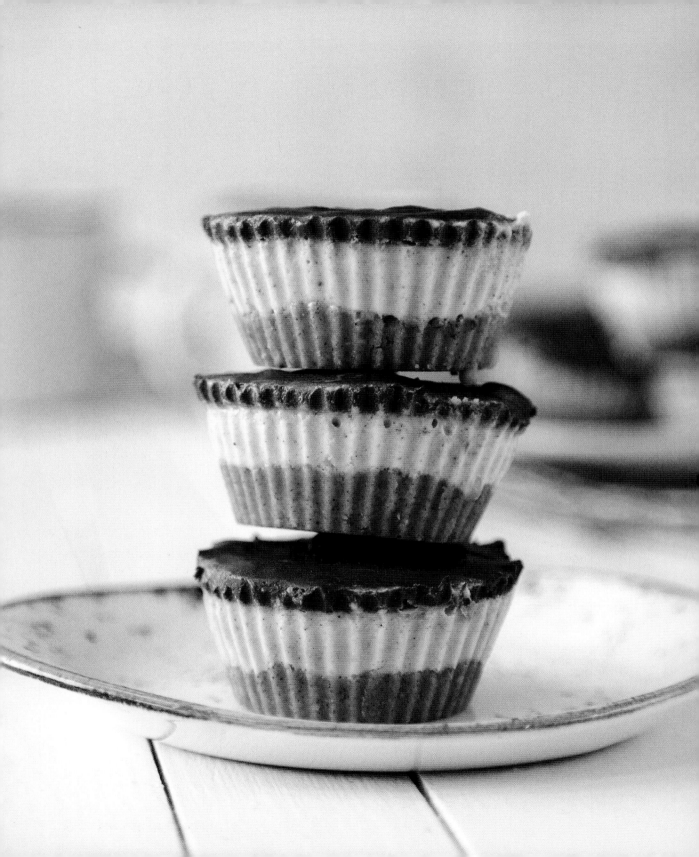

Triple-Layer Frozen Cheesecake Bites

What's the hardest part of making these keto-friendly miniature cheesecakes? Waiting for them to freeze before you sneak a bite. (Stay strong: You can do it!)

MAKES: 6 BITES | HANDS-ON TIME: 15 MINUTES | OVERALL TIME: 15 MINUTES + FREEZING

CHOCOLATE GANACHE LAYER:

2 ounces (56 g) dark chocolate (85% cacao or more)

1 tablespoon (15 g/0.5 oz) butter or coconut oil

2 tablespoons (30 ml/1 oz) heavy whipping cream or coconut milk

ALMOND LAYER:

¾ cup (75 g/2.6 oz) almond flour

1 tablespoon (15 g/0.5 oz) butter or coconut oil, softened

½ teaspoon cinnamon

1 tablespoon (10 g/0.4 oz) powdered erythritol or Swerve, or 3 to 5 drops liquid stevia extract

⅛ teaspoon salt

CHEESECAKE LAYER:

¾ cup (180 g/6.3 oz) creamed coconut milk (page 10), cream cheese, or mascarpone cheese

½ teaspoon vanilla powder, or 1 to 2 teaspoons unsweetened vanilla extract

1 tablespoon (10 g/0.4 oz) powdered erythritol or Swerve, or 3 to 5 drops liquid stevia extract

To make the ganache, break the chocolate into small pieces and place in a small bowl. Heat the butter with the cream in a saucepan over medium-high heat. Once foam starts to develop on top, slowly pour it over the chocolate while stirring, allowing the chocolate and the cream mixture to combine. Set aside to cool.

To make the almond layer, in a bowl, mix the almond flour, butter, cinnamon, erythritol, and salt.

To make the cheesecake layer, in another bowl, mix the creamed coconut milk with the vanilla and erythritol.

To assemble, divide the almond mixture into 6 equal parts and press each part down into a small-medium muffin cup (silicone molds work best). Top each with a dollop of the cheesecake mix, then a tablespoon of the chocolate ganache. Freeze for at least 2 hours before serving. Store in the freezer for up to 3 months.

∽ If your ganache breaks—that is, if the fat separates from the rest of the ingredients—don't panic. Add a tablespoon (15 ml/0.5 oz) of hot water and mix until combined, or place in a blender and pulse until smooth.

NUTRITION FACTS PER SERVING (1 PIECE)

Total carbs: 7.4 g | Fiber: 2.7 g | Net carbs: 4.7 g | Protein: 4.9 g | Fat: 27.1 g | Energy: 277 kcal
Macronutrient ratio: Calories from carbs (7%), protein (7%), fat (86%)

No-Bake Blondie Fat Bombs

My second cookbook features more than one hundred recipes for fat bombs. These nutty, chocolaty blondies are proof that there's always room for more! And since they don't need to be refrigerated, they're ideal for traveling.

MAKES: 16 SERVINGS | HANDS-ON TIME: 10 MINUTES | OVERALL TIME: 10 MINUTES + CHILLING

1½ cups (112 g/4 oz) unsweetened shredded coconut

1 cup (130 g/4.6 oz) macadamia nuts

7.1 ounces (200 g) cacao butter or coconut oil

7.1 ounces (200 g) coconut butter or blanched almond butter

1 teaspoon vanilla powder or 1 tablespoon unsweetened vanilla extract

¼ cup (40 g/1.4 oz) powdered erythritol or Swerve

Optional: ¼ cup (28 g/1 oz) collagen powder

2 tablespoons (28 g/1 oz) cacao nibs or dark chocolate chips (85% cacao or more)

Preheat the oven to 350°F (175°C, or gas mark 4). Spread the shredded coconut and macadamia nuts on a baking sheet. Transfer to the oven and toast for 5 to 8 minutes, or until lightly golden. Stir once or twice during toasting to prevent burning. Remove from the oven and set aside.

Melt both the cacao butter and coconut butter in a double boiler, or a heatproof bowl placed over a small saucepan filled with 1 cup (235 ml/8 oz) of water, over medium heat. Add the vanilla, erythritol, and collagen powder (if using). Mix until combined. Pour the mixture into an 8 x 8-inch (20 x 20 cm) parchment-lined pan or a silicone pan. Spread the toasted shredded coconut and macadamia nuts over the top, and sprinkle with the cacao nibs.

Refrigerate for about 1 hour, or until set and ready to slice. Cut into 4 rows by 4 columns. Keep refrigerated—or store in a cool place at room temperature—for up to a week, or freeze for up to 3 months. (If you use coconut oil instead of cacao butter, be sure to keep the blondies refrigerated or they'll melt!)

NUTRITION FACTS PER SERVING (1 FAT BOMB)

Total carbs: 6.1 g | Fiber: 3.9 g | Net carbs: 2.2 g | Protein: 3 g | Fat: 27.3 g | Energy: 274 kcal
Macronutrient ratio: Calories from carbs (3%), protein (5%), fat (92%)

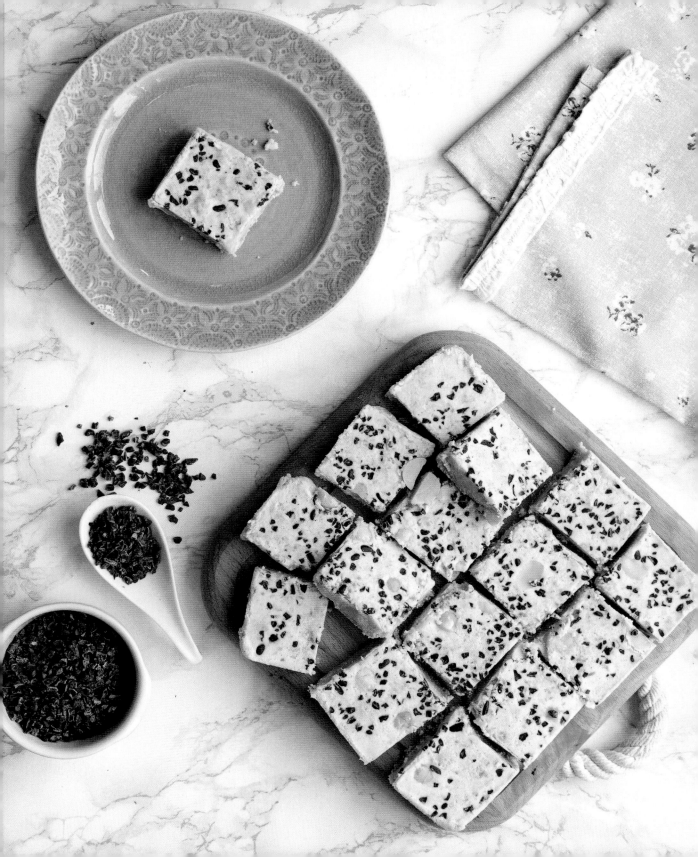

About the Author

Martina Slajerova is a health and food blogger living in the United Kingdom. She holds a degree in economics and worked in auditing, but has always been passionate about nutrition and healthy living. Martina loves food, science, photography, and creating new recipes. She is a firm believer in low-carb living and regular exercise. As a science geek, she bases her views on valid research and has firsthand experience of what it means to be on a low-carb diet. Both are reflected on her blog, in her KetoDiet apps, and in this book.

The KetoDiet is an ongoing project she started with her partner in 2012 and includes *The KetoDiet Cookbook*, *Sweet and Savory Fat Bombs*, and the KetoDiet apps for the iPad and iPhone (www.ketodietapp.com). When creating recipes, she doesn't focus on just the carb content: You won't find any processed foods, unhealthy vegetable oils, or artificial sweeteners in her recipes.

This book and the KetoDiet apps are for people who follow a healthy low-carb lifestyle. Martina's mission is to help you reach your goals, whether it's your dream weight or simply eating healthy food. You can find even more low-carb recipes, diet plans, and information about the keto diet on her blog: www.ketodietapp.com/blog.

Acknowledgments

I'd like to thank everyone at Fair Winds Press who put so much hard work into making all my books happen. Special thanks to Jill Alexander, Renae Haines, Heather Godin, Katie Fawkes, Lydia Finn, Megan Buckley, and Anne Re.

Index

almond butter
  Chewy Pumpkin and Chocolate
    Chip Cookies, 176
  Fat-Fueled Smoothie Two Ways, 162
  No-Bake Blondie Fat Bombs, 184
almond flour
  Cheesy Grain-Free Waffles, 34
  Chocolate Chip Pancakes, 51
  Czech Meatballs with Creamy
    Mash, 149
  Easy Chicken Korma, 114
  Pork Schnitzel with Zesty Slaw, 147
  Quick Salmon Patties, 130
  Raspberry Cheesecake in a Jar, 169
  Tiramisu Mug Cake, 161
  Triple-Layer Frozen Cheesecake
    Bites, 183
almond milk
  Chocolate-Berry Chia Parfaits, 54
  Pork Schnitzel with Zesty Slaw, 147
  Quick Skillet Brownie, 175
almonds
  Crunchy Chile-Lime Nuts, 60
  Key Lime Pie in a Jar, 179
  Pumpkin Pie "Noatmeal," 50
  Quick Keto Cereal, 48
  Skillet Berry Crumble, 173
  soaking, 11
anchovies, in Salmon Niçoise, 97
asparagus
  Bacon-Rubbed BBQ Chicken
    Skewers, 118
  Chicken with Lemon and Tarragon
    Sauce, 109
  Eggs Royale Two Ways, 42
  Pork Stroganoff, 150
Avocado and Kale Pesto
  Broccoli Pesto Salad, 133
  Caprese Stuffed Avocado, 101
  Creamy Broccoli Soup, 87
  Eggplant Parma Ham Rolls, 67
  Green Omelet Wraps, 75
  Hasselback Chicken, 108
  Poached Salmon with Broccoli Pesto
    Salad, 133
  recipe, 19
  Spinach Meatballs with Pesto
    Zoodles, 144
avocadoes
  Avocado and Kale Pesto, 19
  Avocado & Lime Dip, 130
  Beef Fajitas, 140
  Buffalo Chicken Salad in a Jar, 95
  Caprese Stuffed Avocado, 101
  Chimichurri Steak Salad, 105
  Chorizo Egg Muffins, 76
  Fat-Fueled Smoothie Two Ways, 162
  5-Minute Tuna Salad, 99
  Full English Breakfast, 46

  Key Lime Pie in a Jar, 179
  Prawn Cocktail Stuffed Avocado, 102
  Smoked Salmon Chard Wraps, 69
  Tuna Poke Bowl, 129
  Turkey and Chorizo Sliders with
    Guacamole, 122
avoid list, 16–17

bacon
  Bacon BBQ Sauce, 30
  Bacon-Rubbed BBQ Chicken
    Skewers, 118
  baking, 10
  BLT Deviled Egg Salad, 92
  Clam Chowder, 91
  Easy Cauliflower and Egg Hash, 39
  Full English Breakfast, 46
  Green Omelet Wraps, 75
  pan-roasting, 10
  Quick Egg Muffin in a Mug, Two
    Ways, 78
  Ranch Salad in a Jar, 96
  Speedy Cauliflower-n-Cheese, 126
beef broth, for Beef Ramen, 83
beef flank steak, for Beef Fajitas, 140
beef, ground
  Beef Arrabiata Ragu, 143
  Cheeseburger Soup, 84
  Greek Meatball Soup, 88
  Healthy Deconstructed
    Hamburgers, 137
  Quick and Easy Beef Slaw, 106
  Spinach Meatballs with Pesto
    Zoodles, 144
  Taco Frittata, 74
beef rib-eye, for Chimichurri Steak
    Salad, 105
beef sirloin
  Beef Ramen, 83
  Beef Stir-Fry, 139
  Chimichurri Steak Salad, 105
beef stock, for Greek Meatball Soup, 88
berries, mixed
  Blender Berry Ice Cream, 166
  Fat-Fueled Smoothie Two Ways, 162
  Skillet Berry Crumble, 173
blackberries
  Blackberry Lemon Mousse, 170
  Fat-Fueled Smoothie Two Ways, 162
  Skillet Berry Crumble, 173
blueberries, for Skillet Berry Crumble, 173
blue cheese
  Buffalo Chicken Salad in a Jar, 95
  Creamy Broccoli Soup, 87
bok choy
  Beef Ramen, 83
  Good-for-Your-Gut Scrambles, 44
bone broth
  Bacon BBQ Sauce, 30

  Beef Arrabiata Ragu, 143
  Cheeseburger Soup, 84
  Creamy Broccoli Soup, 87
  Middle Eastern Hash, 36
  Pork Saltimbocca, 146
  Pork Stroganoff, 150
  preparing, 13
  Rice Pilaf, 117
  Sausage and Turnip Hash, 38
  Warm Brussels Sprout Salad, 100
Brazil nuts, soaking, 11
broccoli
  Broccoli Pesto Salad, 133
  Chicken with Lemon and Tarragon
    Sauce, 109
  Creamy Broccoli Soup, 87
  Mediterranean Fish Bake, 134
  Moroccan Couscous with
    Halloumi, 125
broccolini
  Chicken with Lemon and Tarragon
    Sauce, 109
  Eggs Royale Two Ways, 42
  Mediterranean Fish Bake, 134
Brussels sprouts, for Warm Brussels
    Sprout Salad, 100
burgers
  Feta Burgers, 155
  Healthy Deconstructed
    Hamburgers, 137
  Turkey and Chorizo Sliders with
    Guacamole, 122

cabbage
  Broccoli Pesto Salad, 133
  Kimchi, 24
  Parmesan-Crusted Chicken Tenders
    with Zingy Green Slaw, 110
  Pork Schnitzel with Zesty Slaw, 147
  Quick and Easy Beef Slaw, 106
carnitas, as Pork Carnitas (a.k.a. Mexi-
    can Pulled Pork), 27
cashews, soaking, 11
cauliflower
  Broccoli Pesto Salad, 133
  Clam Chowder, 91
  Czech Meatballs with Creamy
    Mash, 149
  Easy Cauliflower and Egg Hash, 39
  Speedy Cauliflower-n-Cheese, 126
cauliflower rice
  Crispy Skillet Chicken, 117
  Easy Chicken Korma, 114
  Greek Meatball Soup, 88
  Harissa Chicken Cauli-Cups, 113
  Lamb Kebabs with Tabbouleh, 156
  Moroccan Couscous with
    Halloumi, 125
  preparing, 8

Sardine and Turmeric Nori Wraps, 71
Seafood Risotto, 136
Tuna Poke Bowl, 129
celery
    Buffalo Chicken Salad in a Jar, 95
    Cheeseburger Soup, 84
    Clam Chowder, 91
    Creamy Broccoli Soup, 87
    5-Minute Tuna Salad, 99
    Portobello Tuna Melts, 79
    Ranch Salad in a Jar, 96
chard. See Swiss chard.
Cheddar cheese
    Beef Fajitas, 140
    Cheeseburger Soup, 84
    Cheesy Grain-Free Waffles, 34
    Chorizo Egg Muffins, 76
    Healthy Deconstructed
        Hamburgers, 137
    Portobello Tuna Melts, 79
    Quick Egg Muffin in a Mug, Two
        Ways, 78
    Speedy Cauliflower-n-Cheese, 126
    Taco Frittata, 74
cheesecake
    Raspberry Cheesecake in a Jar, 169
    Triple-Layer Frozen Cheesecake
        Bites, 183
chicken breasts
    Hasselback Chicken, 108
    Parmesan-Crusted Chicken Tenders
        with Zingy Green Slaw, 110
chicken, diced, for Buffalo Chicken
    Salad in a Jar, 95
chicken liver, for Easy Chicken Liver
    Pâté, 65
chicken stock
    Bacon BBQ Sauce, 30
    Beef Ramen, 83
    Cheeseburger Soup, 84
    Chicken with Lemon and Tarragon
        Sauce, 109
    Clam Chowder, 91
    Creamy Broccoli Soup, 87
    Greek Meatball Soup, 88
    Middle Eastern Hash, 36
    Poached Salmon with Broccoli Pesto
        Salad, 133
    Pork Saltimbocca, 146
    Pork Stroganoff, 150
    preparing, 13
    Rice Pilaf, 117
    Sausage and Turnip Hash, 38
    Warm Brussels Sprout Salad, 100
chicken thighs
    Bacon-Rubbed BBQ Chicken
        Skewers, 118
    Chicken with Lemon and Tarragon
        Sauce, 109
    Crispy Skillet Chicken, 117
    Easy Chicken Korma, 114
    Harissa Chicken Cauli-Cups, 113

chile pepper, for Chimichurri Steak
    Salad, 105
chile peppers
    Beef Stir-Fry, 139
    Tuna Poke Bowl, 129
    Turkey and Chorizo Sliders with
        Guacamole, 122
chocolate
    Candied Spiced Cocoa Pecans, 180
    Chewy Pumpkin and Chocolate
        Chip Cookies, 176
    Chocolate-Berry Chia Parfaits, 54
    Chocolate Chip Pancakes, 51
    Fat-Fueled Smoothie Two Ways, 162
    No-Bake Blondie Fat Bombs, 184
    Quick Keto Cereal, 48
    Quick Skillet Brownie, 175
    Tiramisu Mug Cake, 161
    Triple-Layer Frozen Cheesecake
        Bites, 183
chorizo. See Mexican Chorizo; Spanish
    chorizo.
clams
    Clam Chowder, 91
    Seafood Risotto, 136
coconut aminos
    Bacon BBQ Sauce, 30
    Kimchi, 24
coconut butter, for No-Bake Blondie
    Fat Bombs, 184
coconut cream, for Cinnamon Roll
    Soufflé Pancake, 52
coconut flakes
    Pumpkin Pie "Noatmeal," 50
    Quick Keto Cereal, 48
coconut flour
    Cheesy Grain-Free Waffles, 34
    Cinnamon Roll Soufflé Pancake, 52
    Easy Chicken Korma, 114
    Quick Salmon Patties, 130
    Tiramisu Mug Cake, 161
coconut milk
    Blackberry Lemon Mousse, 170
    Blender Berry Ice Cream, 166
    BLT Deviled Egg Salad, 92
    Chocolate-Berry Chia Parfaits, 54
    Cinnamon Roll Soufflé Pancake, 52
    creaming technique, 10–11
    Easy Chicken Korma, 114
    Fat-Fueled Smoothie Two Ways, 162
    Iced Vanilla Latte, 165
    Key Lime Pie in a Jar, 179
    Pork Stroganoff, 150
    Pumpkin Pie "Noatmeal," 50
    Raspberry Cheesecake in a Jar, 169
    Strawberry and Rhubarb Fool, 174
    Tiramisu Mug Cake, 161
    Triple-Layer Frozen Cheesecake
        Bites, 183
coconut, shredded
    Key Lime Pie in a Jar, 179
    No-Bake Blondie Fat Bombs, 184

Pumpkin Pie "Noatmeal," 50
Skillet Berry Crumble, 173
coffee
    Iced Vanilla Latte, 165
    Quick Skillet Brownie, 175
    Tiramisu Mug Cake, 161
collard greens
    Beef Ramen, 83
    Smoked Salmon Chard Wraps, 69
condiments
    Aioli, 21
    Avocado and Kale Pesto, 19
    Bacon BBQ Sauce, 30
    Hollandaise Sauce, 42
    Kimchi, 24
    Mayonnaise, 20
    Pico De Gallo (Fresh Tomato Salsa), 31
    preparing, 13
    Quick Béarnaise Sauce, 23
    Raspberry Chia Jam, 29
    Tartar Sauce, 21
couscous, as Moroccan Couscous with
    Halloumi, 125
crabmeat, for Creamy Crab Dip, 64
crackers, as Speedy Keto Crackers, 62
cream, as heavy whipping cream
    Blackberry Lemon Mousse, 170
    BLT Deviled Egg Salad, 92
    Cheeseburger Soup, 84
    Cinnamon Roll Soufflé Pancake, 52
    Clam Chowder, 91
    Easy Chicken Korma, 114
    Iced Vanilla Latte, 165
    Pork Stroganoff, 150
    Pumpkin Pie "Noatmeal," 50
    Raspberry Cheesecake in a Jar, 169
    Speedy Cauliflower-n-Cheese, 126
    Strawberry and Rhubarb Fool, 174
    Tiramisu Mug Cake, 161
    Triple-Layer Frozen Cheesecake
        Bites, 183
cream cheese
    Cheesy Grain-Free Waffles, 34
    Cinnamon Roll Soufflé Pancake, 52
    Creamy Crab Dip, 64
    Raspberry Cheesecake in a Jar, 169
    Smoked Salmon Chard Wraps, 69
    Speedy Cauliflower-n-Cheese, 126
    Triple-Layer Frozen Cheesecake
        Bites, 183
crème fraîche
    Chicken with Lemon and Tarragon
        Sauce, 109
    Creamy Broccoli Soup, 87
cucumber
    Chimichurri Steak Salad, 105
    My Big Fat Greek Dinner, 155
    Salmon Niçoise, 97
    Smoked Salmon Chard Wraps, 69
    Tuna Poke Bowl, 129
    Tzatziki, 159

dips
    Avocado & Lime Dip, 130
    Creamy Crab Dip, 64
duck eggs, for Southern Duck Deviled Eggs, 59

eggplant
    Eggplant Parma Ham Rolls, 67
    Greek Breakfast Hash, 33
    Mediterranean Fish Bake, 134
    Taco Frittata, 74
eggs
    Beef Ramen, 83
    Blackberry Lemon Mousse, 170
    BLT Deviled Egg Salad, 92
    boiling, 8
    Breakfast Sausage Patties, 35
    Candied Spiced Cocoa Pecans, 180
    Cheeseburger Soup, 84
    Cheesy Grain-Free Waffles, 34
    Chewy Pumpkin and Chocolate Chip Cookies, 176
    Chocolate Chip Pancakes, 51
    Chorizo Egg Muffins, 76
    Cinnamon Roll Soufflé Pancake, 52
    Czech Meatballs with Creamy Mash, 149
    Easy Cauliflower and Egg Hash, 39
    Eggs Florentine in Portobello Mushrooms, 45
    Eggs Royale Two Ways, 42
    frying, 10
    Full English Breakfast, 46
    Good-for-Your-Gut Scrambles, 44
    Greek Breakfast Hash, 33
    Greek Meatball Soup, 88
    Greek Zucchini and Feta Fritters, 81
    Green Omelet Wraps, 75
    Mayonnaise, 20
    Middle Eastern Hash, 36
    Omega-3 Deviled Eggs, 57
    Pizza Frittata, 73
    poaching, 10
    Pork Schnitzel with Zesty Slaw, 147
    Quick Béarnaise Sauce, 23
    Quick Egg Muffin in a Mug, Two Ways, 78
    Quick Salmon Patties, 130
    Quick Skillet Brownie, 175
    Ranch Salad in a Jar, 96
    Southern Duck Deviled Eggs, 59
    Spinach Meatballs with Pesto Zoodles, 144
    Taco Frittata, 74
    Tiramisu Mug Cake, 161

fajitas, as Beef Fajitas, 140
feta cheese
    Beef Fajitas, 140
    Feta Burgers, 155
    Greek Salad, 155
    Greek Zucchini and Feta Fritters, 81

Green Omelet Wraps, 75
Mediterranean Fish Bake, 134
My Big Fat Greek Dinner, 155
fish, marinating, 13. *See also specific fish.*
food list, 15
foods to avoid, 16–17
frittata
    Chorizo Egg Muffins, 76
    Pizza Frittata, 73
    Taco Frittata, 74

garlic
    Aioli, 21
    Avocado and Kale Pesto, 19
    Avocado & Lime Dip, 130
    Bacon BBQ Sauce, 30
    Beef Arrabiata Ragu, 143
    Beef Fajitas, 140
    Beef Ramen, 83
    Beef Stir-Fry, 139
    BLT Deviled Egg Salad, 92
    Breakfast Sausage Patties, 35
    Cheeseburger Soup, 84
    Chimichurri Steak Salad, 105
    Clam Chowder, 91
    Creamy Broccoli Soup, 87
    Creamy Crab Dip, 64
    Czech Meatballs with Creamy Mash, 149
    Easy Chicken Korma, 114
    Easy Chicken Liver Pâté, 65
    5-Minute Tuna Salad, 99
    Greek Breakfast Hash, 33
    Kimchi, 24
    Lamb Kebabs with Tabbouleh, 156
    Lamb Souvlaki with Tzatziki, 159
    Marinara Sauce, 73
    Mediterranean Fish Bake, 134
    Mexican Chorizo, 26
    Middle Eastern Hash, 36
    Moroccan Couscous with Halloumi, 125
    My Big Fat Greek Dinner, 155
    Parmesan-Crusted Chicken Tenders with Zingy Green Slaw, 110
    Pico De Gallo (Fresh Tomato Salsa), 31
    Poached Salmon with Broccoli Pesto Salad, 133
    Pork Carnitas (a.k.a. Mexican Pulled Pork), 27
    Pork Stroganoff, 150
    Quick and Easy Beef Slaw, 106
    Quick Salmon Patties, 130
    Salmon Niçoise, 97
    Sardine and Turmeric Nori Wraps, 71
    Sausage and Turnip Hash, 38
    Seafood Risotto, 136
    Spinach Meatballs with Pesto Zoodles, 144
    Tomato and Sausage Casserole, 152

Turkey and Chorizo Sliders with Guacamole, 122
Tzatziki, 159
ginger
    Beef Ramen, 83
    Beef Stir-Fry, 139
    Easy Chicken Korma, 114
    Kimchi, 24
    Quick and Easy Beef Slaw, 106
    Tuna Poke Bowl, 129
goat cheese
    Eggplant Parma Ham Rolls, 67
    Quick Egg Muffin in a Mug, Two Ways, 78
green beans
    Chicken with Lemon and Tarragon Sauce, 109
    Hasselback Chicken, 108
    Salmon Niçoise, 97
green peppers
    Beef Stir-Fry, 139
    Greek Salad, 155
    Middle Eastern Hash, 36
    Sloppy Joe Lettuce Cups, 121
    Tomato and Sausage Casserole, 152
Guacamole
    Beef Fajitas, 140
    recipe, 122

Halloumi cheese
    Greek Breakfast Hash, 33
    Mediterranean Fish Bake, 134
    Moroccan Couscous with Halloumi, 125
ham
    Eggplant Parma Ham Rolls, 67
    Pork Saltimbocca, 146
    Quick Egg Muffin in a Mug, Two Ways, 78
hash
    Easy Cauliflower and Egg Hash, 39
    Greek Breakfast Hash, 33
    Mexican Hash, 40
    Middle Eastern Hash, 36
    Pork & Radish Hash, 151
    Sausage and Turnip Hash, 38
hazelnuts
    Skillet Berry Crumble, 173
    soaking, 11
hemp seeds
    Pumpkin Pie "Noatmeal," 50
    Quick Keto Cereal, 48
    Skillet Berry Crumble, 173

ice cream, as Blender Berry Ice Cream, 166

jalapeño peppers
    Healthy Deconstructed Hamburgers, 137
    Pico De Gallo (Fresh Tomato Salsa), 31
    Pork Carnitas (a.k.a. Mexican Pulled Pork), 27

jam
    Chocolate-Berry Chia Parfaits, 54
    Raspberry Cheesecake in a Jar, 169
    Raspberry Chia Jam, 29

kale
    Avocado and Kale Pesto, 19
    Chorizo Egg Muffins, 76
    Mexican Hash, 40
    Middle Eastern Hash, 36
    Quick Egg Muffin in a Mug,
        Two Ways, 78
kelp noodles, for Beef Ramen, 83
ketchup
    Healthy Deconstructed
        Hamburgers, 137
    Thousand Island Dressing, 110
keto-friendly food list, 15
Kimchi
    Good-for-Your-Gut Scrambles, 44
    Healthy Deconstructed
        Hamburgers, 137
    recipe, 24
korma, as Easy Chicken Korma, 114

lamb, ground
    Greek Meatball Soup, 88
    Lamb Kebabs with Tabbouleh, 156
    My Big Fat Greek Dinner, 155
lamb leg, for Lamb Souvlaki with
    Tzatziki, 159
lamb shoulder, for Lamb Souvlaki with
    Tzatziki, 159
leftovers, 14
lemon
    Blackberry Lemon Mousse, 170
    Chicken with Lemon and Tarragon
        Sauce, 109
lime
    Crunchy Chile-Lime Nuts, 60
    Key Lime Pie in a Jar, 179
livers, for Easy Chicken Liver Pâté, 65

macadamia nuts
    Avocado and Kale Pesto, 19
    Crunchy Chile-Lime Nuts, 60
    No-Bake Blondie Fat Bombs, 184
    Skillet Berry Crumble, 173
    soaking, 11
mackerel
    5-Minute Tuna Salad, 99
    Omega-3 Deviled Eggs, 57
    Quick Salmon Patties, 130
Manchego cheese, for Chorizo Egg
    Muffins, 76
marinara sauce
    Pizza Frittata, 73
    recipe, 73
mascarpone cheese
    Blender Berry Ice Cream, 166
    Chocolate-Berry Chia Parfaits, 54
    Cinnamon Roll Soufflé Pancake, 52
    Key Lime Pie in a Jar, 179

Tiramisu Mug Cake, 161
Triple-Layer Frozen Cheesecake
    Bites, 183
Mayonnaise
    Aioli, 21
    Avocado & Lime Dip, 130
    BLT Deviled Egg Salad, 92
    Buffalo Chicken Salad in a Jar, 95
    Creamy Crab Dip, 64
    5-Minute Tuna Salad, 99
    Healthy Deconstructed
        Hamburgers, 137
    Omega-3 Deviled Eggs, 57
    Parmesan-Crusted Chicken Tenders
        with Zingy Green Slaw, 110
    Pork Schnitzel with Zesty Slaw, 147
    Portobello Tuna Melts, 79
    Prawn Cocktail Stuffed Avocado, 102
    Ranch Salad in a Jar, 96
    recipe, 20
    Sardine and Turmeric Nori Wraps, 71
    Southern Duck Deviled Eggs, 59
    Tartar Sauce, 21
    Thousand Island Dressing, 110
measurements, 17
Mexican Chorizo
    Mexican Hash, 40
    recipe, 26
    Turkey and Chorizo Sliders with
        Guacamole, 122
mozzarella cheese
    Caprese Stuffed Avocado, 101
    Hasselback Chicken, 108
    Pizza Frittata, 73
    Pork Saltimbocca, 146
muffins
    Chorizo Egg Muffins, 76
    Quick Egg Muffin in a Mug,
        Two Ways, 78
mushrooms, brown
    Beef Ramen, 83
    Beef Stir-Fry, 139
    Good-for-Your-Gut Scrambles, 44
mushrooms, enoki, for Beef Stir-Fry, 139
mushrooms, oyster, for Beef Stir-Fry, 139
mushrooms, portobello
    Eggs Florentine in Portobello
        Mushrooms, 45
    Portobello Tuna Melts, 79
mushrooms, shiitake
    Beef Ramen, 83
    Beef Stir-Fry, 139
    Good-for-Your-Gut Scrambles, 44
mushrooms, white
    Full English Breakfast, 46
    Pork Stroganoff, 150
    Tomato and Sausage Casserole, 152
mussels
    Clam Chowder, 91
    Seafood Risotto, 136

nori, for Sardine and Turmeric Nori
    Wraps, 71

nuts. See individual nuts.

olives
    Broccoli Pesto Salad, 133
    Greek Zucchini and Feta Fritters, 81
    Green Omelet Wraps, 75
    Hasselback Chicken, 108
    My Big Fat Greek Dinner, 155
    Pizza Frittata, 73
    Salmon Niçoise, 97
olives, black, for Taco Frittata, 74
omelets, as Green Omelet Wraps, 75
onions, red
    Buffalo Chicken Salad in a Jar, 95
    Feta Burgers, 155
    Greek Salad, 155
    Mediterranean Fish Bake, 134
    My Big Fat Greek Dinner, 155
    Pico De Gallo (Fresh Tomato Salsa), 31
    Quick and Easy Beef Slaw, 106
    Salmon Niçoise, 97
onions, spring
    Bacon-Rubbed BBQ Chicken
        Skewers, 118
    Beef Ramen, 83
    Beef Stir-Fry, 139
    Creamy Crab Dip, 64
    Easy Cauliflower and Egg Hash, 39
    Kimchi, 24
    Lamb Kebabs with Tabbouleh, 156
    Omega-3 Deviled Eggs, 57
    Parmesan-Crusted Chicken Tenders
        with Zingy Green Slaw, 110
    Pico De Gallo (Fresh Tomato Salsa), 31
    Portobello Tuna Melts, 79
    Quick Egg Muffin in a Mug,
        Two Ways, 78
    Sloppy Joe Lettuce Cups, 121
    Speedy Cauliflower-n-Cheese, 126
    Tuna Poke Bowl, 129
onions, white or yellow
    Bacon BBQ Sauce, 30
    Beef Fajitas, 140
    Cheeseburger Soup, 84
    Chicken with Lemon and Tarragon
        Sauce, 109
    Clam Chowder, 91
    Creamy Broccoli Soup, 87
    Czech Meatballs with Creamy
        Mash, 149
    Easy Cauliflower and Egg Hash, 39
    Easy Chicken Korma, 114
    Easy Chicken Liver Pâté, 65
    5-Minute Tuna Salad, 99
    Lamb Souvlaki with Tzatziki, 159
    Marinara Sauce, 73
    Middle Eastern Hash, 36
    Moroccan Couscous with
        Halloumi, 125
    Pico De Gallo (Fresh Tomato Salsa), 31
    Pizza Frittata, 73
    Poached Salmon with Broccoli Pesto
        Salad, 133

Pork Carnitas (a.k.a. Mexican Pulled Pork), 27
Pork Stroganoff, 150
Portobello Tuna Melts, 79
Quick Salmon Patties, 130
Sardine and Turmeric Nori Wraps, 71
Sausage and Turnip Hash, 38
Seafood Risotto, 136
Sloppy Joe Lettuce Cups, 121
Taco Frittata, 74
Thousand Island Dressing, 110
Tomato and Sausage Casserole, 152
Turkey and Chorizo Sliders with Guacamole, 122
orange juice, for Pork Carnitas (a.k.a. Mexican Pulled Pork), 27

pancakes
Chocolate Chip Pancakes, 51
Cinnamon Roll Soufflé Pancake, 52
parfaits, as Chocolate-Berry Chia Parfaits, 54
Parma ham
Eggplant Parma Ham Rolls, 67
Pork Saltimbocca, 146
Parmesan cheese
Avocado and Kale Pesto, 19
Beef Arrabiata Ragu, 143
Cheesy Grain-Free Waffles, 34
Crispy Skillet Chicken, 117
Greek Zucchini and Feta Fritters, 81
Parmesan-Crusted Chicken Tenders with Zingy Green Slaw, 110
Pizza Frittata, 73
Pork Schnitzel with Zesty Slaw, 147
Seafood Risotto, 136
Speedy Cauliflower-n-Cheese, 126
Speedy Keto Crackers, 62
Spinach Meatballs with Pesto Zoodles, 144
pâté, as Easy Chicken Liver Pâté, 65
pecans
Candied Spiced Cocoa Pecans, 180
Crunchy Chile-Lime Nuts, 60
Skillet Berry Crumble, 173
soaking, 11
pepperoni
Chorizo Egg Muffins, 76
Seafood Risotto, 136
peppers, green
Beef Fajitas, 140
Beef Stir-Fry, 139
Greek Salad, 155
Middle Eastern Hash, 36
My Big Fat Greek Dinner, 155
Sloppy Joe Lettuce Cups, 121
Tomato and Sausage Casserole, 152
peppers, red
Beef Fajitas, 140
Mediterranean Fish Bake, 134
Middle Eastern Hash, 36
Pico De Gallo (Fresh Tomato Salsa), 31

Southern Duck Deviled Eggs, 59
Tomato and Sausage Casserole, 152
peppers, yellow
Beef Fajitas, 140
Mediterranean Fish Bake, 134
pesto. See Avocado and Kale Pesto.
pickles
Cheeseburger Soup, 84
Healthy Deconstructed Hamburgers, 137
Pork Schnitzel with Zesty Slaw, 147
Southern Duck Deviled Eggs, 59
pie, as Key Lime Pie in a Jar, 179
pine nuts, soaking, 11
pistachios, soaking, 11
planning, 14
pork belly, for Pork & Radish Hash, 151
pork chops
Pork Schnitzel with Zesty Slaw, 147
Pork Stroganoff, 150
pork, ground
Breakfast Sausage Patties, 35
Czech Meatballs with Creamy Mash, 149
Mexican Chorizo, 26
pork shoulder, for Pork Carnitas (a.k.a. Mexican Pulled Pork), 27
pork, shredded, for Warm Brussels Sprout Salad, 100
pork tenderloin
Pork Saltimbocca, 146
Pork Stroganoff, 150
provolone cheese
Healthy Deconstructed Hamburgers, 137
Pork Saltimbocca, 146
Portobello Tuna Melts, 79
pumpkin, diced, for Mexican Hash, 40
pumpkin purée
Bacon BBQ Sauce, 30
Chewy Pumpkin and Chocolate Chip Cookies, 176
Chorizo Egg Muffins, 76
Pumpkin Pie "Noatmeal," 50
pumpkin seeds
Quick Keto Cereal, 48
Skillet Berry Crumble, 173
soaking, 11
Speedy Keto Crackers, 62

radishes
Chimichurri Steak Salad, 105
Kimchi, 24
Pork & Radish Hash, 151
ramen, as Beef Ramen, 83
raspberries
Chocolate-Berry Chia Parfaits, 54
Fat-Fueled Smoothie Two Ways, 162
Raspberry Cheesecake in a Jar, 169
Raspberry Chia Jam, 29
Skillet Berry Crumble, 173
rhubarb, for Strawberry and Rhubarb Fool, 174

risotto, as Seafood Risotto, 136
rutabaga, for Cheeseburger Soup, 84

salads
BLT Deviled Egg Salad, 92
Broccoli Pesto Salad, 133
Buffalo Chicken Salad in a Jar, 95
Czech Meatballs with Creamy Mash, 149
Chimichurri Steak Salad, 105
5-Minute Tuna Salad, 99
Greek Salad, 155
Quick and Easy Beef Slaw, 106
Ranch Salad in a Jar, 96
Salmon Niçoise, 97
Warm Brussels Sprout Salad, 100
salmon
Beef Ramen, 83
Eggs Florentine in Portobello Mushrooms, 45
5-Minute Tuna Salad, 99
Poached Salmon with Broccoli Pesto Salad, 133
Quick Salmon Patties, 130
Salmon Niçoise, 97
Smoked Salmon Chard Wraps, 69
sardines
5-Minute Tuna Salad, 99
Quick Salmon Patties, 130
Sardine and Turmeric Nori Wraps, 71
sauces
Bacon BBQ Sauce, 30
Hollandaise Sauce, 42
Marinara Sauce, 73
Quick Béarnaise Sauce, 23
Tartar Sauce, 21
Tzatziki, 159
sauerkraut, for Pork & Radish Hash, 151
sausage
Breakfast Sausage Patties, 35
Full English Breakfast, 46
Sausage and Turnip Hash, 38
Tomato and Sausage Casserole, 152
seeds. See individual seeds.
serrano peppers, for Pico De Gallo (Fresh Tomato Salsa), 31
sesame seeds
Crunchy Chile-Lime Nuts, 60
soaking, 11
Speedy Keto Crackers, 62
Tuna Poke Bowl, 129
shallots
Marinara Sauce, 73
Quick Béarnaise Sauce, 23
shirataki noodles
Beef Ramen, 83
Beef Stir-Fry, 139
shrimp
Prawn Cocktail Stuffed Avocado, 102
Seafood Risotto, 136
sliders, for Turkey and Chorizo Sliders with Guacamole, 122
slow cookers, 13

smoothies, for Fat-Fueled Smoothie Two Ways, 162
soups
    Cheeseburger Soup, 84
    Clam Chowder, 91
    Creamy Broccoli Soup, 87
    Greek Meatball Soup, 88
sour cream
    Beef Fajitas, 140
    Cheeseburger Soup, 84
    Chicken with Lemon and Tarragon Sauce, 109
    Clam Chowder, 91
    Creamy Broccoli Soup, 87
    Ranch Salad in a Jar, 96
Spanish chorizo
    Chorizo Egg Muffins, 76
    Seafood Risotto, 136
spinach
    Avocado and Kale Pesto, 19
    BLT Deviled Egg Salad, 92
    Buffalo Chicken Salad in a Jar, 95
    Chimichurri Steak Salad, 105
    Creamy Broccoli Soup, 87
    Crispy Skillet Chicken, 117
    Eggplant Parma Ham Rolls, 67
    Eggs Florentine in Portobello Mushrooms, 45
    Fat-Fueled Smoothie Two Ways, 162
    5-Minute Tuna Salad, 99
    Full English Breakfast, 46
    Good-for-Your-Gut Scrambles, 44
    Green Omelet Wraps, 75
    Pizza Frittata, 73
    Pork Saltimbocca, 146
    Quick Egg Muffin in a Mug, Two Ways, 78
    Ranch Salad in a Jar, 96
    Salmon Niçoise, 97
    Seafood Risotto, 136
    Spinach Meatballs with Pesto Zoodles, 144
squid, for Seafood Risotto, 136
Sriracha
    Beef Ramen, 83
    Buffalo Chicken Salad in a Jar, 95
    Chorizo Egg Muffins, 76
    Creamy Crab Dip, 64
    Parmesan-Crusted Chicken Tenders with Zingy Green Slaw, 110
    Prawn Cocktail Stuffed Avocado, 102
    Quick and Easy Beef Slaw, 106
    Sardine and Turmeric Nori Wraps, 71
    Tuna Poke Bowl, 129
    Warm Brussels Sprout Salad, 100
strawberries
    Fat-Fueled Smoothie Two Ways, 162
    Skillet Berry Crumble, 173
    Strawberry and Rhubarb Fool, 174
sunflower seed butter, for Chewy Pumpkin and Chocolate Chip Cookies, 176

sunflower seeds
    Avocado and Kale Pesto, 19
    Key Lime Pie in a Jar, 179
    Skillet Berry Crumble, 173
    soaking, 11
sweet potatoes, for Mexican Hash, 40
Swiss chard
    Good-for-Your-Gut Scrambles, 44
    Quick Egg Muffin in a Mug, Two Ways, 78
    Mexican Hash, 40
    Middle Eastern Hash, 36
    Pork Saltimbocca, 146
    Sardine and Turmeric Nori Wraps, 71
    Sausage and Turnip Hash, 38
    Smoked Salmon Chard Wraps, 69
Swiss cheese, for Portobello Tuna Melts, 79

tomatoes, canned
    Bacon BBQ Sauce, 31
    Beef Arrabiata Ragu, 143
    Cheeseburger Soup, 84
    Easy Chicken Korma, 114
    Sloppy Joe Lettuce Cups, 121
    Tomato and Sausage Casserole, 152
tomatoes, cherry
    BLT Deviled Egg Salad, 92
    Caprese Stuffed Avocado, 101
    Chimichurri Steak Salad, 105
    Turkey and Chorizo Sliders with Guacamole, 122
tomatoes, chopped
    Bacon BBQ Sauce, 31
    BLT Deviled Egg Salad, 92
    Caprese Stuffed Avocado, 101
    Lamb Kebabs with Tabbouleh, 156
    Marinara Sauce, 73
    Middle Eastern Hash, 36
    My Big Fat Greek Dinner, 155
    Pico De Gallo (Fresh Tomato Salsa), 31
    Sloppy Joe Lettuce Cups, 121
tomatoes, sliced
    Chimichurri Steak Salad, 105
    Greek Salad, 155
    Healthy Deconstructed Hamburgers, 137
    Mediterranean Fish Bake, 134
    Pizza Frittata, 73
    Portobello Tuna Melts, 79
    Salmon Niçoise, 97
tomatoes, sun-dried
    Green Omelet Wraps, 75
    Hasselback Chicken, 108
tomato paste
    Bacon BBQ Sauce, 30
    Beef Arrabiata Ragu, 143
    Healthy Deconstructed Hamburgers, 137
    Marinara Sauce, 73
    Sloppy Joe Lettuce Cups, 121

tuna
    5-Minute Tuna Salad, 99
    Portobello Tuna Melts, 79
    Quick Salmon Patties, 130
    Salmon Niçoise, 97
    Tuna Poke Bowl, 129
turkey, ground
    Sloppy Joe Lettuce Cups, 121
    Turkey and Chorizo Sliders with Guacamole, 122
turkey liver, for Easy Chicken Liver Pâté, 65
turnips, for Sausage and Turnip Hash, 38

vegetable stock
    Bacon BBQ Sauce, 30
    Cheeseburger Soup, 84
    Chicken with Lemon and Tarragon Sauce, 109
    Clam Chowder, 91
    Creamy Broccoli Soup, 87
    Middle Eastern Hash, 36
    Moroccan Couscous with Halloumi, 125
    Poached Salmon with Broccoli Pesto Salad, 133
    preparing, 13

waffles, as Cheesy Grain-Free Waffles, 34
walnuts
    Crunchy Chile-Lime Nuts, 60
    Skillet Berry Crumble, 173
    soaking, 11
white fish
    Creamy Crab Dip, 64
    Mediterranean Fish Bake, 134
    Quick Salmon Patties, 130

zucchini
    Bacon-Rubbed BBQ Chicken Skewers, 118
    Beef Arrabiata Ragu, 143
    Greek Zucchini and Feta Fritters, 81
    Mediterranean Fish Bake, 134
    Spinach Meatballs with Pesto Zoodles, 144
zucchini noodles
    Beef Ramen, 83
    Pork Stroganoff, 150
    preparing, 8